Large Print Cryptogram Puzzle Book

600 Cryptoquotes about Sports, Movies, Theater, Books, Love, and Music

By JD Leander

Table of Contents

Instructions

Each page contains cryptograms like the one below:

ZYVCV PO DEFX DEV YGSSPEVOO PE FPMV,

ZD FDBV GEI AV FDBVI. -KVDCKV OGEI

Try to determine words and letters based on the patterns of the encrypted letters, then mark the real letters beneath the encrypted ones.

Take a look at the first word in the sample cryptogram above. Whenever there's a five-letter word and the third and fifth letters are the same, it's quite possible the word is either "there" or "where". So, mark the "here" as shown below:

HERE
ZYVCV PO DEFX DEV YGSSPEVOO PE FPMV,

ZD FDBV GEI AV FDBVI. -KVDCKV OGEI

Then fill in the same letters throughout the quote:

HERE   E H   E   E
ZYVCV PO DEFX DEV YGSSPEVOO PE FPMV,
**   E   E   E   E R E**
ZD FDBV GEI AV FDBVI. -KVDCKV OGEI

Continue looking at patterns and relationships between the words and fill in more letters. If you're new at this, then fill them in with pencil so you can erase any incorrect guesses as you learn.

There is one hint for each cryptogram quote in the back of the book. See the Table of Contents for the page number. Each hint looks like this:

K = G

This means that any letter K in the quote is actually a G. There are only two K's in the sample quote on the previous page. Plug them in and you can see the first name for the quoted person is now GE_RGE. I'll bet you can guess what the missing letter is in the first name. Fill it in and then find any other D's in the quote and fill those in.

If you get stuck, the unencrypted quote is in the back of the book. See the Table of Contents for the page number. The unencrypted quote for this sample is:

There is only one happiness in life, to love and be loved. - George Sand

For a free Sample Pack of puzzles, sign up at
https://www.subscribepage.com/samplepack

Cryptograms

1. "BM QVG GMT, BQ'U GDQOS GJJAOQ QVSQ

    UGZSOSQGU S YBMMGO JOAL UGXAMT

    ZCSXG. RIQ YBMMBME QSPGU S CAQ LAOG

    QVSM QVSQ, QAA. BQ UQSOQU YBQV

    XALZCGQG XALLSMT AJ QVG JIMTSLGMQSCU.

    QVGM BQ QSPGU TGUBOG,

    TGQGOLBMSQBAM, TBUXBZCBMG, SMT UGCJ-

    USXOBJBXG. -FGUUG AYGMU

2. "CIS BHQZ H ZIW? D LHQ UWZ CIS H ZIW,

    PWEDWKW TW. ZAWXW HXW BHCO, FSFW." -

    BHEZWX OIPLAHJ, ZAW PDU EWPIBOJD

3. "DAJWODZ XWA ZESRFA CBZX ECDBJXOSX

    AFACASX ES COZXAJESR XWA XAHWSEMQAZ

    OSK XOHXEHZ BN JOHESR EZ AGDAJEASHA.

    TQX BSHA IBQ WOPA XWA NQSKOCASXOFZ,

    OHMQEJESR XWA AGDAJEASHA EZ O COXXAJ

    BN XECA." -RJAR FACBSK

4. "EVI JHBBPTMB VTLI T KITQCM EVTE RTM

    KPQI CHE EKC VHMNJIN IPDVEO EVCHBTMN

    TGIJPRTMB. EVTE QHEB EVIG IWTREYO EIM

    OITJB UIVPMN VCKTJN RCBIYY." -JIN BGPEV

5. "F EFUN DKQFO," QTN QBFP QEHGEL,

"CNOBKQN GTNR F TNBM FI, F . . . F EHQN

DLQNEV GFITFR DLQNEV, FV ITBI DBUNQ BRL

QNRQN. F CNOHDN NDWIL BRP VKEE BEE BI

HRON, BRP F OBR VNNE ITN GTHEN NBMIT

MHFEFRZ BMHKRP DN." — QBMBT S. DBBQ,

ITMHRN HV ZEBQQ

6. "FVQHVJNPUC UN Q GQWWVJ DM PQOUEX

CVDCFV FDDY QW ZDS QEH XQUE

LDEMUHVELV, NVVUEX PDR ZDS JVQLW. UM

ZDS'JV UE LDEWJDF, WPVZ'JV UE LDEWJDF." -

WDG FQEHJZ

7. "GM PVC'O GKC VO ZDTM. GM PVC'O GKC DC OZM JDVW. VB UMCMJVH TVCVUMJ, K YIBO PVC'O EKUIJM DIO GZMJM MHBM OD QHVA." - QVO GKHHKVTB

8. "IGNKOUVFX OU E ITEUU XSW VEQN OJ GOMG UIGSST SF ISTTNMN, PGNFN XSW DOMWFN SWV VPS CTWU VPS OU 10, SF USKNVGOJM." - BNJJOU FSBKEJ

9. "IJ RBR NBT BXABJT SBYVNS IQ SNQTQ AHDRT: WBDQ BOR TNBDQ. SNBS'T ANJ AQ EYS HO WXPOPWT. SNQ HOXJ SNPOV P WBO RH PT SDJ SH VPUQ KBWG. PL PS AHDGT, PS AHDGT." -SPVQD AHHRT

10. "JECVQJNTDJRGE UCV NS GJ KRSD T PFZ

KTIOJ CUU QRS WCFVQ TDB ZCF VSTIIZ

WTD'Q QSII KRSQRSV RS KCD CV ICJQ KRSD

RS WTVVGSJ RGNJSIU KGQR EVGBS SGQRSV

KTZ." -MGN WCFVGSV

11. "JGTMGIE DVJ ETZWVMZEME EDZJ MNDM

FIWDAZVK MNW HGQI-LZVQMW LZRW XDE

ZLSGEEZFRW, MNDM GVW XGQRJ JZW ZV

MNW DMMWLSM. MNQE, XNWV Z KGM QS HIGL

MNW MIDTA DHMWI TGRRDSEZVK DM MNW

HZVZEN RZVW, Z HZKQIWJ Z XDE JWDJ." -

IGKWI FDVVZEMWI

12. "K JYF'O HVYC QBKFP DYZ. K PR RGO OABLB YFZ AYUB MGF. KO'E Y PYDB, YFZ OAYO'E ARI K YD PRKFP OR OLBYO KO." -WBF PLKMMBC TL.

13. "TVJ DKOX NV MX KMCX NV SXANXU TVJUHXCE, NV CXN KCC VE TVJU XGVNLVAH YV. WVA'N XOXU EVUYXN NDKN TVJ FCKT ZLND TVJU HVJC KH ZXCC KH TVJU MVWT." - RKUXXG KMWJC-PKMMKU

14. "VRD SHGGDQDOJD WDVTDDO VRD UBS

WKBBNBKZDQ KOS VRD ODT WKBBNBKZDQ

HM VRD EDQMDZ. VRD UBS WKBBNBKZDQ

JKQDS KWUFV VRD OKAD UO VRD GQUOV.

VRD ODT WKBBNBKZDQ JKQDM KWUFV VRD

OKAD UO VRD WKJX." -MVDLD IKQLDZ

15. "VS ZERKTZH RCK CT E BJGNRK JU

HNKBCUCB EXKEH." QK ZJJI E VJGZQUGR JU

MKKX. RJJICTY EXJGTF ZQK ICZBQKT, LKT

HECF, "C'V MKZZCTY QJGHKIKKNCTY CHT'Z

CT ZQK ZJN ZKT." -V.E. XJMMCTH, ZQK

EDEIKTCTY

16. "YHQX OXHOMX EXMKXUX LHHNEPMM KY P

QPNNXG HL MKLX PAR RXPND. K'Q UXGJ

RKYPOOHKANXR CKND NDPN PNNKNIRX. K

SPA PYYIGX JHI KN KY QISD, QISD QHGX

KQOHGNPAN NDPA NDPN." -EKMM YDPAZMJ

17. "ZPF RDGHFT ZW ZPF OBZLYRZF SOFGZLWD

WJ BLJF, ZPF ODLUFTGF, RDK FUFTVZPLDC

LG...42!" -KWOCBRG RKRYG, ZPF

PLZEPPLIFT'G COLKF ZW ZPF CRBRMV

18. "ZP'J IHP PCB MZJKEZDZPA PCKP MBTZIBJ

AHO; ZP'J CHL AHO MBKD LZPC PCB

SCKDDBINBJ PCB MZJKEZDZPA UXBJBIPJ

AHO LZPC. LB CKWB KI HEDZNKPZHI PH PCB

KEZDZPZBJ LB MH CKWB, IHP PCB

MZJKEZDZPA." -FZY KEEHPP

19. 'DRCOB! CRIH KH DRCOB!' VXW BOH

VPEZDHWW LEG PN KG WPJD, XFZ BOH

DRCOB PN DPIH WOPFH PF KH RF BOXB IHEG

OPJE. -OHDHF QHDDHE

20. "...ON MDF PCSPQG DC YSNPFMNII. IDTN PSN

ODSM YSNPF, IDTN PKLQNUN YSNPFMNII,

PMG IDTN LPUN YSNPFMNII FLSZIF ZHDM

'NT." -BQEEQPT ILPXNIHNPSN, FBNECFL

MQYLF

21. "A CDDH AJBD BFZAY ZGZV, VFRHZ BFZAY

FRJE, LRB BFZAY PRWH, RJE TAVF BFZK

CSWH, PSB A RK BFAJHAJI, 'A RK IDAJI BD

PSYG GDS." – VZOZ PRCCZVBZYDV

22. "A TLEHVU HK RVH HIV BLEO ZXPZVU BKW HIV OVFKEU ILJB, OK A OVEH HIAO HTVVH:

"EVVU HTK PKWV UXESO KE IKPV FKXWH BKW HIV DVOH FWKTU VGVW!

#DLQJKWELHAKE." – DWAHHEVQ RWAEVW

23. "AKJ NTLA ENBTQAFMA AKEMW EM AKJ TIVNBEG WFNJL EL MTA XEMMEMW SRA AFYEMW BFQA; AKJ JLLJMAEFI AKEMW EM IECJ EL MTA GTMZRJQEMW SRA CEWKAEMW XJII." —BEJQQJ UJ GTRSJQAEM, CFAKJQ TC AKJ NTUJQM TIVNBEG WFNJL

24. "AKUZ EXXH GXLLUI KDOOUZG, S ESQU

CKDZPG TXI CKU RSIDLWU DZH S HXZ'C ESQU

D HDRZ AKSLK CUDR XI LXNZCIV OUITXIRG

SC." -UHNDIHX EDWUDZX

25. "ANK XTLM IN FN ZNDMIXYGC YG ANKU SYEM

IXTI YZ XNGNUTPSM TGF GNI WNOTUFSA YE

ANK TUM IN SYLM YG QMTWM OYIX

ANKUZMSE." – STUUA PUNOG

26. "AUN KCNNYW JNBTNXNE AUHA TA SHW H VTATMND'W ELAP AR SHAVU H OBHP. TA SHW H YTDE RI SRCY TD AUHA TA CNZLTCNE HAANDATRD, GLEKQNDA, OHATNDVN, HBB AUN WRVTHB XTCALNW." -ATQJNCBHYN SNCANDJHYNC

27. "AXDPRAF RL KQKM SMKNKDKMIRAKN. RD'L J VXALDJAD MKIRANKM DX ZXMY PJMN, LDJU CXVHLKN JAN AKQKM EKTRKQK DPJD UXHM CHDHMK RL JLLHMKN." – DRI VJPRTT

28. "B NVWZV IWZMS WDO B NVWS MWVI, OWS

WXVIZ OWS, SIWZ WXVIZ SIWZ. BV VRRY HI 17

SIWZN WDO 114 OWSN VR TIURHI WD

RLIZDBKEV NFUUINN." – MBRDIM HINNB

29. "B RCURDT LPCC EBST, DQY ZRKP LUQ PDPT

RMS QMP JQYLZ. EPPF LUQ QFPM RMS QMP

OCQTPS. DQY MPKPW CPRWM RMDLZBMI BA

DQY'WP LZP QMP LRCEBMI." – IQWSBP ZQUP

30. "BEA GMEPR YUA NBR RIUKMFUNRIX PUAOUI

GMEPR MC NBR NMODB DOX EL VEPNOFRA.

VEPNOFRA BUGR TUJR NBRT UII IESR NBUN."

— FUXTMLJ PBULJIRF, NBR KED AIRRV ULJ

MNBRF LMGRIA

31. "BIDB WZIPNU (CWZANLD VP. CZWVUP) OUWF FBU WNLU 'KYL'F CZWV ZWW AYIP ZQIJUJ [YO WZLDIZDU ICYL VU]' EZJ CYJJNQWA FYY PIKU. 'NF'J NL FBU QYYH,' N JZNK. BU KNKL'F BNF VU." — UVVZ FBYVCJYL

32. "BJMJK PHMJ QY, BJMJK PHMJ HB, LBW VSJB NSJ QYYJK SLBW HO DQKO, XLZ VJ SLMJ NSJ LRHGHNZ ND SLBWGJ NSJ VHB VHNS NSJ WHPBHNZ NSLN VJ LRODKRJW NSJ GDOO." - WDQP VHGGHLXO

33. "BLEN LM I GPNIGSN MNG LY VPLDP GPNSN ISN WKG ENV XSIDGLDIWBN NYGSIYDNM." — TLDGZS PKRZ, BNM OLMéSIWBNM

34. "BQV WQTW BOM MHO'U XDNN RHIKXDNZ XWHKU. SOHC UWBU RHI'KD ABGBJND. IOMDKXUBOM UWBU B NHU HZ GDHGND JBUUND CQUW B NHU HZ UWQOTX – MDGKDXXQHO, JHMR QVBTD HK CWBUDPDK DNXD – XH SOHC UWBU QU'X OHU LIXU RHI. RHI'KD OHU BNHOD." – WHNNR WHNV

35. "BTVYV IYV OVYBIFX RIKFO PLIEFBFVK IXC OTIYIOBVYFKBFOK SWL'GV DWB BW TIGV. XLURVY WXV: SWL'GV DWB BW TIGV I JFEE BW JFX." – RWR YFOTIYCK

36. "BZQFF ZGSLQFL DSL FVPZBM TDBOZFU D MFDQ. DSL V XRNFL VB. V ORGXLS'B PFB FSRGPZ RY VB." – QVO YXDVQ VS BR WF BZF TDS

37. "C OBSYGB Y DNNQ FCWSTBJ MTBE C RWNFFBQ WJLCED WN GYIB WTBG GCRR WTB OYPP YEQ RWYJWBQ WJLCED WN GYIB WTBG TCW CW." – RYEQL INAUYZ

38. "C OVMM OBV GCFU, UPWVYPFZ'U DPOOX SCR, UPWVYPFZ'U DPOOX MPUV. TNUO FPR'O JCDBO XYPNO CO. TNUO OAZ OP DVO YVOOVA." -ZPDC YVAAX

39. "C'OD QKIADM UKK REIM EPM UKK FKPJ UK

FDU EPXURCPJ LUEPM CP URD QEX KS VX

JKEFL. C QCFF PKU FDU VX UDEVVEUDL

MKQP, EPM C QCFF PKU FDU VXLDFS MKQP." -

VCE REVV

40. "CA IVHHXJ WAM IEUW DAE'LX MAC, CA

IVHHXJ WAM IVCD TVIXK, CA IVHHXJ WAM

IVCD UWVIOGACKWGOK, CA IVHHXJ WAM

IVCD KEOXJ SAMNK, DAE'JX CAH MGCCGCT

CAM, KA DAE KHGCY." -SGNN OVJUXNNK

41. "CB OXSNY XLK MLUDKO, CB WSOJKLY XLK MNKKQSOJ, CB XLCY XLK HUZKLKQ ASPG PGK AKNPY NKWP MB PGK VXAY UW BUFL JFXLQY—MFP S XC X EFKKO!" — YUVGUHNKY, XOPSJUOK

42. "CFI FUQJIVC VXDBB CA UOYHDQI DT CFDV VZAQC DV CFI ATI NFIQI MAH OASZICI UBB AHC, RDLI DC UBB MAH FULI, UTJ MAH UQI VCDBB RICCDTR EIUC TA SUCCIQ NFUC MAH JA. NFIT MAH FULI CFI XDBBIQ DTVCDTOC CA KDRFC CFQAHRF CFUC, DC DV LIQM VZIODUB." – IJJDI QIIVI

43. "COGI T YTBDH KWVG PI HPNB, T CWD

ZUWRTIE YPB VPIGR. IPC T'V ZUWRTIE HP CTI

EPUY HPNBIWVGIHD WIS HOG VPIGR TD VPBG

HOWI T GFGB SBGWVGS T KPNUS VWQG." –

WIITQW DPBGIDHWV

44. "CPFXC X KFPYUD XY BF JY, XDV BF GJTT

PFRXJD XY BF JY. CPFXC BJR XY BF NUHTV

OF, XDV BF GJTT OFNURF GBXC BF YBUHTV

OF." -LJRRZ LUBDYUD

45. "CQCPJ ANH GPKBVH UMC YKPDH YMK LDGJI

IKRRCP YGVUI UK WC LCDC. N MGQC G

SPCGU PCILKVINWNDNUJ UK IMKY UMCF

VKU OBIU MKY UK WC DNAC G IKRRCP

LDGJCP, WBU MKY UK WC DNAC G FGV." –

LCDC

46. "CT ROU NRRG GUUG CO LSS JB SCTU C GCG,

C GR HUVUOW CW THRJ JB ZUHB QRPS." —

ICSSCLJ QFLAUQVULHU

47. "CWNL NQ UJRCIMWMZ. NU RWZ GWQU W RNLXUJ, IM WL AIXM, IM W HWZ, IM W ZJWM, YXU JPJLUXWGGZ NU KNGG QXYQNHJ WLH QIRJUANLT JGQJ KNGG UWDJ NUQ CGWSJ." — GWLSJ WMRQUMILT

48. "CXAAXAE XU KOM QGUK XQVGWKHAK KOXAE XA QB RXPM, HPKMW FWMHKOXAE. FWMHKOXAE PXWUK, CXAAXAE AMSK." - EMGWEM UKMXAFWMAAMW

49. "D LUAUT CDC XKM RFKR MNZ GKL'R IU K

LDGU EZM KLC BDL. D XKDC RFKR DJ D BKX

HQKMDLE RFDTC IKXU KLC SM SNRFUT

TNZLCUC RFDTC BDRF RFU BDLLDLE TZL, D'C

RTDH FUT ZH." -QUN CZTNGFUT

50. "D OIDSC IZ KGMCZ IDB JNTZ DS OIZ JDGBO

FENV MJ OIZ RNXZ, NSH OIZS IZ RMO

BQGRZGV NO INEJ-ODXZ NSH TNXZ KNTC OM

JDSDBI OIZ RNXZ NSH OIZV AMS." —

XNGBINAS EVSTI

51. "D VG OW RSODKB; D EKBL MWFQSY CVFY NDQS GU WLCSF LSVGGVLSB, VOY D ZSNDSHS VNN GU LSVGGVLSB XVO MDO LCS LDLNS VB LCSU MWFQ CVFY, LWW." – NDO YVO

52. "D'QJ ZAS I SUJAEC SUIS DB CAM ZDQJ 100% IKK AB SUJ SDNJ, VANJUAL SUDFZV LDKK LAEY AMS DF SUJ JFH." –KIEEC TDEH

53. "DE ZQS'XH SIDGW UTKE ZQSX VQGVHGNXTNDQG NQ KQQB GQXYTK, NUHG ZQS'XH QGKZ UTKE CTZDGW TNNHGNDQG NQ MUTNHJHX HKIH ZQS'XH LQDGW." — YTWGHNQ

54. "DH NDNS'H XMHHVY GKMH JTUHMOIV GMU

DS QYJSH JQ BU, GV'N MIGMRU OMYYR JS HJ

HKV VSN. 'QJZVU SVLVY WBDH' DU HKV

UIJFMS MTJLV HKV HBSSVI MH HKV CDSF

AJGVY UHMNDBX, MSN GV QJIIJGVN HKMH

HJ HKV IVHHVY." – EMXDV LMYNR

55. "DIKIL WGFSPLI TGJL RGKI BAGLT AG ACGBI

TGJ VPAWC ZD FGKZIB. ACIT'LI VLZAAID HT

BWLZSAVLZAILB, TGJLB ZB VLZAAID HT

NGQ." — IXLID SIDPXRGLZQP UL.

56. "DN, ACS HCG'U MGCL IJ, RSU N DWVVJG UC RJ IWOONJH UC UDJ IWG LDC YCGUNGSJK UC OSHJBA NGUJOOSVU ACS JTJOA ULC INGSUJK." — RJG HNUIWOK, UJG INGSUJK NG DJWTJG

57. "DP OCC WTZ JML BDMLWK ML WTZ VDXCI, KTZ TOI WD VOCG MLWD EMLZ AOKORCOLAO" — TSEUTXZN RDJOXW

58. "DQZN EJNC XFNGRLIN. EJN RGCN XFNGRLIN EJNM JGZN YJNK EJNM YGUN LX SIBC G KQDJECGIN." — GFSINW JQEAJABAU

59. **"DRS UKM K DSKQ TXKMC KC K URZXS VSDSPQBYSC BDC CAJJSCC. MZA QKM RKFS DRS IPSKDSCD NAYJR ZG BYVBFBVAKX CDKPC BY DRS UZPXV, NAD BG DRSM VZY'D TXKM DZISDRSP, DRS JXAN UZY'D NS UZPDR K VBQS." – NKNS PADR**

60. **"DTQNTBJCFYBCFQY FJ QYK QS CZK EQJC NQEEQY BYI IKBIPFKJC QS IFJKBJKJ BYI FCJ CQPP QY JHNNKJJ BYI ZBDDFYKJJ FJ ZKBLX." – UBXYK RTKCVWX**

Copyright © 2019 by Cottage Street Press, All Rights Reserved

61. "DWDFE LOFQ GDDCY H XOJ ST RVONYE JS

FDNOGC VDF JVHJ QOTD OY H LHND HGC

OJ'Y HQQ HXSKJ VHWOGL TKG." — PHGCHPD

VHWDGY, JHBD OJ QOBD H WHNU

62. "DWFRNL QRBB DVUN AWT PVDWTL;

MNBNFRLRWI QRBB DVUN AWT GRSE; OTM

MENVMGN QRBB DVUN AWT HWWJ." —

MNGGNISN DVII

63. "DZDCIHBD BQ WJI CIDWJ SO ZBTIHD. BW BQ

WJI UIAL SEESQBWI SO EDQQBST. OBNH BQ

TSW WJI DAW SO QZJSNDAQ, KXW SO

BNNBWIADWIQ." — YIATIA JIARSM

64. "E IFO UMFGK AVKTGELZPA VKT IMPPK

AVKTGELZPA. EO'A PEOZPM XPMW KPG

LZPPAP FM XPMW FJT HPVO." - FALVM

HVTEAFK, OZP FTT LFYRJP

65. "EAJ'OX FATTG SGNX IA FA ISOAJFS SXQQ.

BAOCX ISGT GTE TLFSIHGOX ISGI EAJ'NX

XNXO VOXGHXV. WJI LT ISX XTV, EAJ PTAB

EAJ'QQ WX ISX ATX CIGTVLTF. EAJ PTAB

BSGI EAJ'NX FAIIG FA. VA LI. VA LI!" —

GZAQQA KOXXV

66. "EB E DIAQNJ YSYX JEY, PAJ BAXLEJ, NYR

RIED LY FO YHERGHI: RIY AKNO HXAAB IY

KYYJYJ BAX RIY YZEDRYKTY AB PAJ UGD

FQDET" — VQXR SAKKYPQR

67. "EBOQP'O KVLKRO AGGT MGKVVR

PKJIKMJQP. QJ'O JIG AGOJ HMBD SNM EG JN

DGJ KLKR SMNE JIG GUGMRHKR

FMGOOBMGO CBOJ SNM K OGPNTH UQK K

DNNH ONTD." – UQVVG UKVN

68. "EHK'D PSWLCJS ZHCJLSYR OZ GTWD ZHC

TWFS WXXHPBYQLTSE, OCD OZ GTWD ZHC

LTHCYE TWFS WXXHPBYQLTSE GQDT ZHCJ

WOQYQDZ." – NHTK GHHESK

69. "EMV UJHS PC B TYVVH JG B EMJHN EP CVBW. B TYVVH JG YGVS EP NJAJHN ZPUUBHSG, HPE PDVIJHN EMVU; BHS MVW WBNV PHZV WPYGVS JG MBWS EP BLLVBGV."
— VYWJLJSVG

70. "EPB GJS NSMDV TNBFGBKHL (NT) NSMDSEDVK DKMGJENL PSJ EGNKBM UVCRDB CVYDBJ DKEV NBSQDEL." — JEBYBK CSOBB, EVZDH BQBHENDHDEL

71. "ERA FDH BTJCBW ZJTFX JR ERAW VRDIZ, RW ERA FDH OAZJ VR JCWRAVC JCB PRJTRHZ DHG WBZJ RH ERAW ZJDJAZ. KAJ TJ'Z DII DKRAJ QRWX." – XWTZJTHB ITIIE

72. "EW EJC BHJNFCN REUXCD SBCFC'D EJC SBLS XD WLXF, EJC SBLS'D OEEN LJN JXJCSZ-CXOBS SBLS LFC UCFZ MLN. REDS REUXCD DSLFS MLNGZ LJN DSCLNXGZ OCS PEFDC." — QBLFGCD MHIEPDIX, SBC GLDS JXOBS EW SBC CLFSB VECRD

73. "F LKUNM NPNAR GFJEUN DB UAKFJFJQ, OEU F XKFM, 'MDJ'U WEFU. XEBBNA JDC KJM VFPN ULN ANXU DB RDEA VFBN KX K TLKGSFDJ.'" -GELKGGKM KVF

74. "F RHY'M ALY WIWO XAHQ W EBWSSNYKN

VNEWLJN F WQ WXAWFR. FYJMNWR, F ALY

MHIWAR FM VNEWLJN MBN HYSO IWO MH

NJEWCN XNWA FJ MH MAWQCSN FM

VNYNWMB OHLA XNNM." —YWRFW

EHQWYNEF, KHSR-QNRWS KOQYWJM

75. "F'I L ANRMMW CHHK JFGGRN. F'I L

MRNNFUZR ZHPRN. LGK F NQU FM FG

ANRMMW CHHK JYRG F JFG." -MHI UNLKW

76. "FEN IALF TN KQS EACN WAH VL FA KHNQFN

   FEN MNLF CALLVMON KASJVFVASL WAH

   LYKKNLL, FENS ONF PA AW FEN AYFKAIN.

   FEN HVJN VL Q OAF IAHN WYS FEQF TQZ." —

   CEVO RQKDLAS

77. "FEUSU MSU AMWJ HSUUW PSMHZWD GW

   FEGD VZSRP ZK VMJDGPU GWWD, UNUW MD

   FEUSU MSU AMWJ VEGFU EMSFD, SUP

   RGZWD, DGRUWF VZAUW MWP ZFEUS

   GWTSUPGYRU FEGWHD..." — VGRRGMA EUWSJ

   EIPDZW

78. "FJJSI GAM NJBTVI, YPVC GOV AJY NVOV

VAYVOYGTANVAY. YPVC IDIYGTA NV GAM

PVKX NV WJXV ETYP NC OVGK KTUV." —

GOKGTAG YTFVAISC

79. "FOI FG CMI LTIRCIKC IDSITVIOQIK VO EVGI

VK RQMVIZVOL SITKFORE LFREK CMRC

FCMITK KRVY NFAEY WI, 'VJSFKKVWEI CF

RCCRVO.' WI STFAY FG XFAT KAQQIKK ROY

KMRTI XFAT KCFTX NVCM FCMITK." – TFWITC

QMIIUI

80. "FRH XHYEFR GU N UDXS CRGBXJ PH

JDZHVFXI ZHXNFHJ FG FRH HYJBZNYVH GU

FRH RBSNY PXNJJHZ." — NXUZHJ

RDFVRVGVT

81. "FZYNX NY LEO TGOWLOYL XSFFZRNXWLNSR

NR LEO VSGCU. OMOR NP AOSACO USR'L

ZRUOGYLWRU LEO CWRTZWTO LEWL HSZ'GO

YNRTNRT NR, LEOH YLNCC JRSV TSSU FZYNX

VEOR LEOH EOWG NL." – CSZ GWVCY

82. "G KXO NSSQ VSRVMS WXMM GQ MRES GQ

UREGSN, BRR, XQO WSMB GQ MRES WJRU GB.

XQO G KXO NSSQ VSRVMS OGS GQ UREGSN

XQO GB NSSUSO URJS JSXM BKXQ OSXBK GQ

JSXM MGWS." — FKSMNSX UXJBGQ, BKS

JSXMMT WCQQT BKGQP XIRCB XVXBKT

83. "G PMQI MWCMZE AFGIY AB TI AFJI AB

XZEIWS, AB UGHV APBEI TMAAWIE G SIWA

CIFI GXUBFAMRA. XZ JWAGXMAI

FIEUBREGTGWGAZ GE AB XZEIWS. G HBJWY

RIQIF TI MRZAPGRK IWEI." -MFAPJF MEPI

84. "GDC XQE'R QSUQGH XDERODS

XTOXCWHRQEXFH. NDUFZFO, GDC XQE

QSUQGH XDERODS GDCO QRRTRCLF,

QKKODQXN, QEL OFHKDEHF. GDCO DKRTDEH

QOF RD XDWKSQTE DO RD SDDM QNFQL QEL

BTPCOF DCR NDU RD WQMF RNF HTRCQRTDE

JFRRFO." — RDEG LCEPG

85. "GDCKC'R UCSCK QUJ GCMMAUH ZDQG

JLW'MM RQJ LK VL UCPG, CPICFG GDQG AG'R

ELWUV GL EC RLXCGDAUH QRGLUARDAUH.

EJ HLV, RAK, JLW QKC Q IDQKQIGCK." — YLDU

DWRGLU, GDC XQMGCRC BQMILU

86. "GIL OCEWNL W PWQQ SWEL GK FA

NIWQCHLT, WR OTC PILT GILA IOEL KQAFBWN

OZBWHOGWKTZ, PWQQ XL GK SK RKH WG." —

VLHHW POQZI, SKQC-FLCOQ XLONI

EKQQLAXOQQ BQOALH

87. "GIVSCJVQIW, WDG ZJEQ VD KDV ADUUW

JHDGV MQDMIQ VZSKBSKL WDG NZDGIX

ZJEQ MIJWQX ZSC XSYYQUQKVIW. WDG'UQ

VZQ DKQ MIJWSKL VZQ MJUV ND SV ZJN VD

HQ WDGUN." — QAJK CRLUQLDU

88. "GK OSI GXSG GXHOH AHW TSMJ GXHMB OXMRRMWPO GK ESGQX GEHWGI-GEK XMBHRMWPO LMQL S NSRR MO AHBHRI GK OSI GXSG S YMKRMW MO EKKJ SWJ QSGPFG, SWJ GXSG XSARHG MO OK AFQX TSTHB SWJ MWL." -VKXW NKIWGKW TBMHOGRHI

89. "GP'K XEWT PN UIEP E DIWKNC MXN CIFIW SGFIK YD." "XIWNIK SIP WIVIVUIWIT, UYP HISICTK CIFIW TGI." –UEUI WYPX

90. "GRT XKUQTOLT FOSZC GRT GPKGR, GRT ZSPYU QC CQNHYT. QG'C NQCTPXMYT, CSYQU XYY GRT ZXA GRPSKER. MKG QV ASK LSKYU VSSY GRTN, TBTO VSP X CTLSOU, GRTO ASK LXO NXFT GRTN ZSOUTP, XOU GRTO ASK ESG GS CTT CSNTGRQOE PTXYYA CHTLQXY." — LRPQCGSHRTP OSYXO

91. "GWVK QPPEN CP BLOIB ON ILK GOIIOIB, THK KWP SHPNK RLX XPVYWOIB ELKPIKOVJ OI CFNPJR VN V YLVYW VIZ CF QOZN VN ZOAPXN. OK'N KWP EHXNHOK LR PDYPJJPIYP." – XLI L'TXOPI

92. "HFS AOG FEP?' LTP ZEMBR LTXEKU GFEKUL

ZEMB 'HFS AOG FEP?' EG WBPEKRBR FEP SD

QBEKU T MER TKR HTGAFEKU VWELSK

PSJEBL, HFEAF EL VWSQTQZX HFX

VWELSKBWL GTZMBR ZEMB GFTG, GSS." —

GSR USZRQBWU, GFB WBDSWPBR

93. "HKFIR, MPRFPGQPLJ, XOVM DKVA, CKOQ

RJZZPLC OLM, KH FKIVRJ, ZXJ ZXVPQQ KH

HPLOQQT OFXPJWPLC TKIV CKOQR. ZXJRJ

OVJ OQQ QJRRKLR PL QPHJ." —AVPRZP

TOSOCIFXP, CKQM-SJMOQ HPCIVJ RAOZJV

94. "IAPU YWZIPMA VL JFAQ DWZ BQWJ DWZ'IA

UVYBAO NAHWIA DWZ NAMVQ, NZR DWZ

NAMVQ PQDJPD PQO LAA VR RFIWZMF QW

KPRRAI JFPR." -FPICAI UAA, RW BVUU P

KWYBVQMNVIO

95. "IBNL WTBWFT QJAT MW GMNL ZCTO LCTE'KT

DSBML LB DHCJTAT NMHHTNN. LCTE PMJL

BO LCT BOT EDKU FJOT. LCTE QJAT MW DL

LCT FDNL IJOMLT BY LCT QDIT BOT YBBL

YKBI D ZJOOJOQ LBMHCUBZO."– KBNN

WTKBL

96. "ICDIUUISDI WY SNM X YWSFTUXV XDM GTM X EXGWM. LNT XVI ZEXM LNT RN VIAIXMIRUL."

    – YEXBTWUUI N'SIXU

97. "IHQ LC, YXOOXOE XFO'S FHLCSTXOE STVS TVRRCOF FNPPCOKJ HO STC IXCKP YTCO STC YTXFSKC UKHYF VOP STC BQHYPF QHVQ. YXOOXOE XF FHLCSTXOE STVS UNXKPF RTJFXBVKKJ VOP LCOSVKKJ CWCQJ PVJ STVS JHN SQVXO VOP CWCQJ OXETS STVS JHN PQCVL." -CLLXSS FLXST

98. "IJIKO TIFKGY SLK F YIKL WQTV XIBHE PHVY TLWIVYHEB PYHGY IJIKO YIKL KIRQHKIT - F JHMMFHE." — KLXIKV VLPEI, WHTTHLE: HWULTTHXMI

99. "IMMBOUNN TY U YTRKNL VURL; 22 RLF GXUYL U OUNN IMQ 90 RTFDBLY UFC UB BXL LFC, BXL VLQRUFY HTF." -VUQW NTFLSLQ

100. "IMUSRI RTJFQTI DUE FQJSJFRTS, PR RTJFQTI DUE RU MKJD OD RQT SEKTI, PR RTJFQTI DUE RU HZUV VQJR PR LTTKI KPHT RU VPZ JZA KUIT-PR RTJFQTI DUE JOUER KPLT." – OPKKPT YTJZ HPZB

101. "ISNXMIB MO ARPUC-PIL-GXMND, DFUDWN ESV

GMIIMIB PIL RSOMIB, PIL TPQAD NXPN'O GXQ

WDSWRD BVPJMNPND NS NXPN OS TKUX." –

ONDJD IPOX

102. "IXYYXYJ XZ YRD T ZRSVDXSV DGXYJ; XD'Z

TY TFF DXSV DGXYJ. KRP URY'D IXY RYWV XY

T IGXFV, KRP URY'D UR DGXYJZ CXJGD RYWV

XY T IGXFV, KRP UR DGVS CXJGD TFF DGV

DXSV. IXYYXYJ XZ GTLXD. PYMRCDPYTDVFK,

ZR XZ FRZXYJ." -AXYWV FRSLTCUX

103. "J HCJTX HCJN JN QCU LYYJN HMMX NM

OBTU OMGJTE AJFHZWLN MV ZN. PLFBZNL

CL XTLQ HCBH ALMAYL FMOL JT BTS MZH MV

UMZW YJVL, BTS B AJFHZWL VJRLN HCLO JT

HCL OMOLTH HCLU WLBFC MZH HM UMZ." —

KZ GJTFLTH, HCL YZFXU AYBFL

104. "J'CS KRF R NDP DM FGRYORXTV RBF

VSPORXTV JB UA XRGSSG, OHP BD URPPSG

YKRP RBADBS VRAV RODHP US, J'U

FSPSGUJBSF PD OS PKS OSVP VTJSG JB PKS

YDGNF, RBF BD DBS JV IDJBI PD VPDE US." —

NJBFVSA CDBB

105. "JFAO Q FZE LFZL ZLLZNV ST MDAGXSUQU -

FA ZUVAE RA JFZL JZU LFA RZLLAX JFAO Q

NZRA IZNV. Q UZQE MDAGXSUQU - FA

LFSGWFL LFZL Q UZQE IDGA XSUAU! US

LFZL'U JFZL FA ZDJZKU NZDDAE RA ZTLAX

LFZL. JFAOAHAX FA UZJ RA, FA'E FSDDAX,

"FADDS, IDGA XSUAU!" — LAOOAUUAA

JQDDQZRU

106. "JFZTX TZ Q CVDFO, BPJCPVQJPLBQH

JTZBVPZZ. NTKP UPV BUP BTJP QLO

QBBPLBTDL ZUP OPZPVKPZ, QLO ZUP TZ

SDFVZ. ZHTNUB UPV QLO BUPVP GTHH XDJP

Q OQS GUPL SDF XQHH QLO ZUP GTHH LDB

QLZGPV. ZD T IPNQL ZHPPCTLN HPZZ BD

NTKP UPV BUP BTJP ZUP LPPOPO." -CQBVTXY

VDBMFzz

107. "JI JZ IWRI DJES FB IWJEDJEU IWRI JZ IWP

HMFKQPV; IWRI VFGJPZ, GJSPF URVPZ RES

IWP JEIPMEPI, SPGJOPZ IWRI ZJVHQX RVNZP

IWP JVRUJERIJFE RMP VFMP JEIPMPZIJEU

IWRE LWRI R QJKMRMX ZIFODZ." — Z.R. IRLDZ,

IWP ZHJMJI FB JVRUJERIJFE

108. "JKHC DBVDGB PKC A'J RQB ZBPR MVJBH'P

PVLLBX DGKCBX AH RQB MVXGW. A WVH'R

RQAHS PV. KHW ZBLKTPB VO RQKR,

PVJBWKC A ITPR JANQR ZB." -JAK QKJJ

109. "JNFVF OIB GF QFXQTF JNIJ NIUF OXVF

JITFYJ JNIY BXA, GAJ JNFVF'P YX FCKAPF

SXV IYBXYF JX MXVH NIVLFV JNIY BXA LX." –

LFVFH WFJFV

110. "JQU JDSU MQUT JQUVU DI TB BTU JQUVU JB

PUUG IBVVE PBV EBO BV JB HQUUV PBV EBO

DI MQUT C KGCEUV DI SCRU." – JDS ROTHCT

111. "K'CF PQN ZR VFQML ZR OKWPZ QVV US VKOF

– WRZ ZR VFQML ZR XFFY JUKVKLW. KO SRE

JUKVF ZPKLWJ IKVV IRMX REZ." – JFMFLQ

IKVVKQUJ

112. "KLPUSA SFBLMASB ZFQXFRSB UBSXA CO

NZRRUFI RESK UFRL ARLMO TLMK XFB

MSALJPUFI RESK ZN RESMS LF RES AGMSSF.

RES ILXJ QXA, XA XJQXOA,

UBSFRUTUGXRULF, CZR XJAL MSJUST." —

YSXFUFS CXAUFISM, U BL XFB U BLF'R: X

EUARLMO LT KXMMUXIS UF RES KLPUSA

113. "KN CYJ LCCU UJJU KY EII GV IKNJ K UKU, K

UC QJMJYA KA NQCG GV DJQV WCRI." —

TKIIKEG WZEHJWMJEQJ

114. "KW VTCMVTZZ TWL KW VACKWMCC, UBMEM TEM UBEMM UONMC DJ NMDNZM. UBDCM SBD RTGM KU BTNNMW, UBDCM SBD STUQB KU BTNNMW, TWL UBDCM SBD SDWLME SBTU BTNNMWML." – UDRRO ZTCDELT

115. "KXYV YT FIWKRSXSG. YF WXG CXTF X WYVPFI, RS XV MRPS, RS X HXG, RS X GIXS, EPF IBIVFPXCCG YF ZYCC TPETYHI XVH TRWIFMYVJ ICTI ZYCC FXDI YFT KCXOI. YA Y NPYF, MRZIBIS, YF CXTFT ARSIBIS."– CXVOI XSWTFSRVJ

116. "L JNKNA RASKNX ELRYVGR DZ BLSAZ. VJN HYVGXB SXESZH YSKN HVDNRYLJM HNJHSRLVJSX RV ANSB LJ RYN RASLJ." — VHWSA ELXBN, RYN LDQVARSJWN VT ONLJM NSAJNHR

117. "L'KS BJUBNO HSJE PXOLW LO ECS FMJN UBN EF ZLKS BM LMOEBMEBMSFXO PFPSME ECS HSSJ FH OJFU PFELFM. EF QFPBMELWLOS LE BMT ZJFQLHN LE BMT ZLKS LE B OFXMTEQBWD BMT B QCNECP." – EBNJFQ OULHE

118. "L'RS PLXXSV PJBS IFYU 9000 XFJIX LU PZ

QYBSSB. L'RS DJXI YDPJXI 300 CYPSX. 26

ILPSX, L'RS NSSU IBGXISV IJ IYOS IFS CYPS-

TLUULUC XFJI YUV PLXXSV. L'RS HYLDSV

JRSB YUV JRSB YUV JRSB YCYLU LU PZ

DLHS. YUV IFYI LX TFZ L XGQQSSV." –

PLQFYSD AJBVYU

119. "LCNZB FEUMB/LEAXEM: E GBCK ZEM LB

EMUKMB, BRBM E XEM VKWMT PKXBAGWMT

EP PWXQYB EMV CBEPPNCWMT EP QNAAWMT

E ZKEA KM E UKNMT LKU'P PGKNYVBCP AK

YBA GWX IMKF AGEA AGB FKCYV GEVM'A

BMVBV." — ZGCWPAKQGBC MKYEM

120. "LGWHPYL KRL SHCWPWJVJKX CZ XCIH

JGGJMLMK ELPKR....PME UMCQ KRLHL JN

MCKRJMT J YPM EC KC NPBL XCI." —

NIFPMML YCVVJMN, KRL RIMTLH TPGLN

121. "LQ HAVLO XM WYM QEER EQ KEGM, DKJF EB,

PLGM HM MNOMVV EQ LW; WYJW

VACQMLWLBP, WYM JDDMWLWM HJF

VLOUMB, JBR VE RLM." — SLKKLJH

VYJUMVDMJCM, WSMKQWY BLPYW

122. "LQHBEELWYX LE RJEN T WLI KBVM NSVBKD

TVBJDM WC EQTYY QXD KSB PLDM LN

XTELXV NB YLFX LD NSX KBVYM NSXC'FX

WXXD ILFXD NSTD NB XZHYBVX NSX HBKXV

NSXC STFX NB USTDIX LN. -QJSTQQTM TYL

123. "M TAAW QE M UHMVZ JKZDZ SR DZMHQPR,

ZEVMUQES, KAUZ, CZEUMQD, HALZ MGC

CZMPK HQZ." — GQWQPM CBCMGQ

124. "MH JKZ'DT QKMFQ RK ABVJ VR VBB, JKZ'DT

KZR RK YMF. NVOTNVBB, NKVDI QVGTO,

ABVJMFQ STKAVDIJ, M UVRT RK BKOT." -

ITDTE STRTD

125. "MIR OFXKMOPDG IDO OXPRMIZGV OFRYZDJ ZGOZUR XH IZP MIDM MDCRO XARK ZG UZHHZYNJM OZMNDMZXGO. Z SDO UKZARG XG QW MIR UROZKR, MIR FDOOZXG, MIR HRRJZGV, DGU MIR FKZUR XH QRZGV D HXXMQDJJRK." – DGUKR ZGZROMD

126. "ML UMQQP WK LE QEPK. MY M'W H LBEZCQKWHUKB, HAV M VEA'L LOMAU LOHL WT LKWJKB WHUKP WK EAK, LOKA ML'P CKGHZPK M GHA'L PLHAV QEPMAX. LOHL'P LOK SHT M HW HCEZL SMAAMAX, HQQ M KFKB SHALKV LE VE SHP YMAMPO YMBPL." - RHGUMK BECMAPEA

127. "MLIM'H VLIM MLW EKNYWH XK. MLWR XKA'M

WAMWCMIYA ZH, MLWR XKA'M HWAX MLW

EWHHITW: 'VW FICW.' MLWR TYNW ZH GYAWH

MK HIR, MLWR IHHYTA ZH JICMH: UKLA

VIRAW, MLWXI DICI, HLYCGWR MWEJGW,

MIQW RKZC JYFQ." — FKAAYW VYGGYH,

CWEIQW

128. "MRTUTHTX OPN KTTC CDFT GXDWDGDYDUQ

EUOPUT ... INVW XTLTLATX WREW ECC WRT

STPSCT DU WRDV MPXCB REHTU'W REB WRT

EBHEUWEQTV WREW OPN'HT REB." -K.

VGPWW KDWYQTXECB, WRT QXTEW QEWVAO

129. "MWBI XWB PLIJ LG HVIXUVFFBJ EIJ GQLULX EFLKIBJ MLXW QAUQVGB, XWB RVJN LG HEQERFB VZ GV PAHW PVUB XWEI MB UBEFLSB." — ULHW UVFF

130. "MXMLA HTJM T ZMUH EZEA T ZEB VMYMTXTUS JA JIJ. T'V HMPP KML T ZEB SITUS HI BYKIIP CWH T'V CM IWH IU HKM BHLMMH DPEATUS NIIHCEPP. T EPZEAB KEV E CEPP IU JA NMMH." -LIUEPVI

131. "N DL MGNQENPR D YNBJ, DPE JKJBX EDX N IBDNP, N DEE LABJ YGJQ. DI HGVI ISJ BNRSI LALJPI, N QNRSI ISJ LDIZS." —LND SDLL, RAQE-LJEDQ VAZZJB TQDXJB

132. "N JONME N'H LYFLAB BZ HXVO HZQD OLTTA FNJO SZZEB LMR HZGNDB LMR BJXCC. N JONME N WDJ HZQD DKVNJDR LSZXJ FDYY-RZMD QDTQDBDMJLJNZMB ZC YNCD JOLM YNCD NJBDYC. - VDYNMD" — QNVOLQR YNMEYLJDQ, SDCZQD BXMQNBD & SDCZQD BXMBDJ: JFZ BVQDDMTYLAB

133. "N LCY PTDS COCNXYM KNXG CXZ KRDKIT

LWTX N LCY SJRXO, ATHCRYT MWTS LTDT

ONDIY' HJIJDY. ARM MWCM LCY JXIS

ATHCRYT N ZNZX'M LCXM KTJKIT MJ LDNMT

UT JVV VJD LWCM N HCX ZJ. LWTX N OJM

NXMJ US 20Y, N ZTHNZTZ MWCM LCY

YMRKNZ." – ZCXNHC KCDNHG

134. "N XLSR RZ KQ L OLO, WNJUR LSO WZJQDZUR.

N XLSR RZ KQ L VZZO WLRBQJ. N'HQ UEQSR

UZ DPYB ZW DT GNWQ ZS RBQ DZHQ LSO

RJLHQGGNSV LJZPSO RBQ XZJGO RBLR APUR

RZ UQR PE L BZDQ WZJ DT WLDNGT LSO KQ L

VZZO OLO NU UZDQRBNSV RBLR DZRNHLRQU

DQ." – JNYFT EZSRNSV

135. "NGB ABU PX HQN NGB FPZZ NQ FPH.

BRBSUOQJU GMX NGMN. PN PX NGB FPZZ NQ

ESBEMSB NQ FPH NGMN PX PLEQSNMHN." –

OQOOU AHPVGN

136. "NMYBWGCGCQW JBMXGJ HXW BTHPWK

YHCVTP MV H ICQW-HVK-H-SHTI CVNS

NMRXG, GSW JBHNW EWGAWWV PMRX

WHXJ." – EMEEP FMVWJ

137. "NXLI W QOLA JI OXVO SVQHLOSVMM YJGUO,

W'K OXWIHWIC VSJGO SVQHLOSVMM, W'K

OXWIHWIC VSJGO NWIIWIC – SGO OXLUL'Q QJ

KGYX OXVO CJLQ WIOJ OXJGCXO VSJGO XJN

W'K CJWIC OJ JALI OXWQ CVKL GA OJ

JOXLUQ. WO'Q QJ KGYX KJUL OXVI BGQO

SVQHLOSVMM." -YVUKLMJ VIOXJIF

138. "O MIKGW VNENA FREN LIJJNV HRMY OVJI QU MRANNA TOJFIKJ JFN KVWUOVL CKDDIAJ IP QU FKCHRVW, TFI TIAYC PKGG JOQN RJ R CJANCCPKG XIH!" – GOVWCRU WRENVDIAJ

139. "O MVOUBKCT KH HCUYCTY PVC LCYH TCN HYNNJY SCQ NVON LOI'H BQOMNKMY, NVON LOI'H MCUBYNKNKCT, NVON LOI'H BYQSCQUOTMY. NVYI OQY OJPOIH HNQKDKTW NC AY AYNNYQ. NVYI LCT'N JKDY KT NVY BOHN." – AQKOTO HMGQQI

140. "OC LAKLEWU PW GE TE EZUK GSUKU FVM GE WUU PB P NFV RUUL QKPVTPVT WLEKGW. P'O SELPVT PG ELUVW MEEKW BEK AW." – MUVVPW KEMOFV

141. "OCFAF DAF ZKPX OBZ ZQOLZKI AFHDAULKH RZEELOEFKO. XZW'AF FLOCFA LK ZA XZW'AF ZWO. OCFAF LI KZ IWRC OCLKH DI PLTF LK-MFOBFFK."– QDO ALPFX

142. "OI XSB CYVZF JZ DMCR BTUNZ ECTXC OY CPSBR, O DSBNF YCX CPSBR CY JBUM CY O UCT RCVZ." — KSPZKR LCKNCTF

143. "OLHP RPLRSP OZD C IZWP ZJJCJNYP –

HZDMP C YL...MNJ C JICVA DLN IZWP JL. DLN

IZWP JL MPSCPWP CV DLNGOPSX BIPV VL LVP

PSOP YLPO – JIZJ HZAPO DLN Z BCVVPG

GCUIJ JIPGP. "– WPVNO BCSSCZHO

144. "OMPZPOHSZ, OMPZPOHSZ, OMPZPOHSZ.

WGZJH, JSOIDU PDU HMGZU...LS LSZS

RZSHHX ZVJHX GDGHGPYYX. LMSD XIV MPAS

P QZSPT WIZ P WSL LSSTJ XIV BSH P QGH IW

ZVJH." – BZPMPC MSDZX

145. "OW'D MCHHZ ARS WAQ FRBRPD RM WAQ

PQTB SRPBV RHBZ DQQJ PQTBBZ PQTB SAQH

ZRC STWFA WAQJ RH T DFPQQH." — THWARHZ

YCPXQDD, T FBRFISRPI RPTHXQ

146. "OX'K IVX YBMX M JVWON OK MSVDX, OX'K

BVY OX OK MSVDX OX." — HVPNH NSNHX

147. "OXTZJO QZDCJDO C YTVR YDJUDDV

QTVJDAXTZCZMDO JGCJ BCOJO C

BMSDJMAD. MJ CBOT HMNDO PTWZ BMSD

OJZWQJWZD, RMOQMXBMVD CVR C

HDVWMVD, OMVQDZD, XWZD SWBSMBBADVJ

JGCJ SDU TJGDZ CZDCO TS DVRDCNTZ

XZTNMRD." -YTY QTWOP

148. "OZDKWCFXL EC CBW BFLBWTC YWMWY FT XZC EIZSC AFXXFXL. FC'T EIZSC KHWKEHECFZX, OZSHELW, SXGWHTCEXGFXL EXG XSHCSHFXL VZSH KWZKYW, EXG BWEHC. AFXXFXL FT CBW HWTSYC." -QZW CZHHW

149. "P JBU'A QFLD APED RBW QBHHPDI. FA AQD DUJ BR AQD JFX, P AWDFA EX KBH FI F QBHHX. PA'I IBEDAQPUC P YBLD JBPUC." - JFLPJ HDMVQFE

150. "P VIPBU NPBGQX, QAEPGJ, XBM QXTPN IXEG XWZXOJ HGGB NWAJGWO XJJANPXVGM. VIG EGSO GXSWPGJV LGALWG ZIA QXMG KPWQ ZGSG QXTPNPXBJ." — KSXBNPJ KASM NALLAWX

151. "PCFUIYB GN ZGJB FUGIOUGIGIV U YUP. GR ACH WC U VCCW SCM CR GO, ACH DGZZ UZDUAN LUQB U WBXBIWUMZB EHGBO PGWB." — O.P. DUZZUYB

152. "PEHYW YH LOO LADEF FBLYUYUI YU KLBPDUV, FBLYUYUI FD EUXSBHFLUX LUX EHS PEHYWLO SUSBIV CDB DEB IBSLFSB TOSLHEBS AV LFFEUYUI FD FKS ULFEBLO OLMH DC FKS EUYJSBHS." – ZLUS HYASBBV

153. "PNNLW DIC YNEBRW DFR WKQJ CBOORFRIG RIGBGBRW GJDG B ORRM BG'W PRWG GN MRDER QDWGBIS GN GJR QDWGBIS CBFRQGNFW. GJRT JDER D ODF PRGGRF BCRD NO HJDG GJRT'FR CNBIS GJDI B HNKMC." — DMBWGDBF QFNWW

154. "PXOGK VSG'I HXBS CESG HNSI GXC CQOHP NG CESNQ ESFQCI, MOC NG CESNQ SPSI." - UNHHNFV IEFWSIASFQS, QXVSX FGR YOHNSC

155. "QEO POCGQRSGB QERMT CPYGQ RQ RH QECQ MY QLY VRDOXQYDH YD CXQYDH LYDI QEO HCWO LCJ. JYG CBHY BOCDM MYQ QY PO CSDCRV YS VRHXGHHRYM CMV XYMSBRXQ."
— OLCM WXTDOTYD

156. "QEZ SBI NCQI RBTD IYQJJQIYE UQS KB XBD RBT. QEZ NCQI RBT UQS KB XBD RBTD IYQJJQIYE." – JQLVU FBCSEBS

157. "QGGU HPFS VSGKRZ KCNYG. FMVGSZAKMV AP KWXNGYG KMHAXNME SGBFNSGZ DKNAX KMV IGCNGD NM HPFSZGCD, YNZNPM, XKSV JPSQ, VGAGSRNMKANPM, KMV VGVNWKANPM. SGRGRIGS KCC AXNMEZ KSG UPZZNICG DPS AXPZG JXP IGCNGYG." -EKNC VGYGSZ

158. "QT XKK VYHT OLYH CUT PXHT RAIW YO OXHAKATP, CUXC PCLFJJKTW XIW OYFJUC. XIW AO BYF DLAIJ CYJTCUTL STYSKT QUYPT HTICXKACATP XIW TGSTLATIVTP XLT CUT PXHT, QUYPT YDPTPPAYIP XLT PUXLTW, BYF UXNT X DAJ XWNXICXJT." – KFAP PFXLTM

159. "QTEKA EYMMYZHWH 6 UKX FQH QYIQHXF-
IJNXXYAI ENSYH NB FQH XTEEHJ KAW
JHFTJAHW AYVQNMKX VKIH FN NXVKJ-
UYAAYAI XFKFTX." — V.G. QKGKJW, ANF YA
FQH HRH

160. "QXNC XR H GXRTHRT. PYTB XS XBQTESR
UAZI WNAAGRSITHC, XS SHFTR AMTI HR SYT
BZCWTI ABT YAICABT; XS WARRTR SYT
TBDUCTR; GXITESR SYT LXBTHN KNHBG;
LNHUR XHKA SA UAZI LRUEYT. HR PXSY
YTIAXB, SYT HBSXGAST SA QXNC XR CAIT
QXNC." — QIHBF EHLIH

161. "R HATQ RP IWQD ZAJ SA PA KQQ

KAYQPWRDS, ODN ZAJ QDPQL OK OD

RDNRTRNJOH, ODN ZAJ HQOTQ OK O SLAJU.

CQXOJKQ ZAJ'TQ OHH CQQD CAJDN

PASQPWQL CZ PWQ KOYQ QFUQLRQDXQ." —

PAY WRNNHQKPAD

162. "R XJWEKF'I ORAH CJW IXJ UHFIY LJS ZEE

CJWS LZFUC SWEHY RL MHDRFK IDHP IDHC

KRKF'I DZAH Z ERIIEH MRI JL GEZRF

JSKRFZSC HAHSCKZC BRFKFHYY, ZFK Z

ERIIEH EJJBRFO JWI LJS IDH JIDHS LHEEJX,

IJJ." — YRKFHC MWUDPZF

163. "RK KOLU PINIP, QLKO UE DRHV ZOVULFRP KRPIHKU RPP FRZRXPI EB JELHC KOI URDI KOLHCU, KOI DIHKRP ULJI QRU KOI UIZRARKEA." – JLAW ORVOSAUK LH XLCCIA KORH KOI CRDI

164. "RNQDDP KPTAR HXSX YVEXVLXG KTSLPA LD CYEX KTSXVLR TV XTRA DKKDSLBVYLA LD GXODVRLSTLX LQXYS KSYDSYLYXR." — NTPEYV LSYPPYV, TMDBL TPYNX

165. "RO RM IEO PIELJS OE FRMAEXPD OSP

MPADPO EU T CKTH, ROM OSELJSO TIF

UPPKRIJM—OSP TAOED WLMO YP TYKP OE

AEIXPDO OSPW RIOE KRXRIJ OPDWM." —

NEIMOTIORI MOTIRMKTXMNR, ADPTORIJ T

DEKP

166. "RZCW WVMQQ VZQX ZNAFV OU NMD EGMVH

WTPFCTGMH, EGMTG NHTZOH MTACMT MC

MVW AEC PMDGV. M QAJHL VGZV

WTPFCTGMH ZCL MVW QMVVQH WKZPXQHW

VGZV KHDDU DQFHL AC GHPWHQR. EMVGAFV

OU WTPFCTGMH, M EAFQLC'V GZJH RHQV

PHZLU VA TAOKHVH." — WGZCCAC OMQQHP

167. "RZZO NQBWJ BTW CWPCWC NPM BTW

CZIPMC FYRR RZZO NQBWJ BTWXCWRHWC" —

RWFYC DNJJZRR, NRYDW YP FZPMWJRNPM

168. "SCEA QGHBM NU SGTJU ACEI NULIW

LFFGTAEB? EIM JALBB CEPLIW AG NUCEPU

NK ACU THBUJ?" — TEFUEH VBEAUU

169. "SFBP ZTV CYXN ZTV NBYAP CATD JFB

DXIJYWBI ZTV DYRB YPR XJ DTJXQYJBI ZTV

JT STAW BQBP FYARBA." – PYJYNXB OVNLXI

170. "SJRR OL QRN-MJADEQPLN, GTC CDL ADJVL

QM XJCLW EA J CQTW NL MQWSL.

OJNNLPEPY. DLJWCMLRC. AESF. PQACJRYES.

JP QNL CQ CQNN OSSJWCDZ, JWPQRN

YRJAAOJP, JPN ACTJWC AJOTLRA'

NQSTOLPCJWZ MERO, HEAEQPA QM REYDC.

GZ JRR OLJPA, CJFL J GQX." — J.F.

FTZFLPNJRR

171. "SJUKBS DM HNP-HDTKB. CK EZVCUK. QJVK

DM VJB-HDTKB. CK HFJSKQZU. GNBGKDS DM

MKUQ-HDTKB. CK GJFKQZU." – WNEB

XNNPKB

172. "SPISXP YWP XPAA LZVOJ UI YSSXYZM RIZ YA RIZ HWIT IXMPW. XVNP AUYWUA IZU TVUC PQPWRIKP OXYSSVKH TCPK RIZ UYJP Y SII YKM HIPA MITKCVXX NWIF UCPWP." -AXIYKP OWIAXPR, V TYA UIXM UCPWP'M GP OYJP

173. "SPQUXTQVPA LKV WTH QL EUQA QWVHV ELLB HLSPH CWL NKLC VRVBA HVMBVQ TZLSQ CBUQUKI, GUBVMQUKI, GVHUIKUKI, EBLGSMUKI, TKG TMQUKI ZSQ TBV HQSMN UK QWLHV XUHVBTZPV GTA OLZH CBUQUKI BVRUVCH. CUPP HLXVZLGA WVPE QWVX, EPVTHV?" — GTRUG URVH

174. "SUJQDXA UO XMM EDQHUMPO XM JQ JPDUQV UI JMMFO. RQI OTMPSV TMSV UX PE UI CDMIX MC XTQR QZQDA OUIKSQ VLA MC XTQUD SUZQO LIV OLA, 'U'R CDQQ'." — OUVIQA JPHTRLI, CDLIF HLEDL'O RD. ORUXT KMQO XM GLOTUIKXMI

175. "SVYL XURW NFPSUWFLA, IZVSLNLW SZL CVX HL, PZLWFAZ SZLC, RAL SZLC, HRS KUO'S ALSSTL DUW SZLC." – CFV ZVCC

176. "T NGY KGUIZJE COZJY AGULZUQTKN 90% ZL YPG YTQG. YPGUG'E CHVCBE YPCY HTYYHG EGHL-FZJOY, OJY T FZK'Y HGY TY NGY YZ QG." – YZUUTG VTHEZK

177. "T PKTOL JA UGHFPHNP RTMPYGA ZFN

HRHGA PTJH T ZFVLHC YDP PKHGH, T UFRH

TP HRHGAPKTOU T KFC. T VHXP

HRHGAPKTOU YDP PKHGH. PKFP'N ZKFP T'J

JYNP QGYDC YX." -ITJJA MYOOYGN

178. "T VPUTG FW RUPH VW LUEI FDPI XUTBDPI

HWIFG'V RUYYIG. TX T HW IAIPOVRTGC T

JUG, UGH PDG UF XUFV UF T YWFFTQBO JUG

UGH FWLIWGI FVTBB QIUVF LI, T HWG'V

VRTGE WX VRUV UF XUTBDPI." – LUPTWG

SWGIF

179. "T'Z TU HVWFLJQ LQBKFRQ T'Z UWVZKJ KUX RJTDNHJO KVVWDKUH. K JWH WG SQWSJQ XWU'H JTMQ HNQZRQJAQR KUX T NKSSQU HW LQ HWHKJJO TU JWAQ ITHN ZORQJG." – ZTMQ HORWU

180. "TI TQ NRNW CSN XWSXAW IS EW RQJWU IFW OLWQITSM GFTYF XLIQ IFWD QOLRNWAB TM CNSMI SC IFWDQWAZWQ" — RNIFLN DTAAWN, IFW YNLYTEAW

181. "TUTMZ VBQTREMZ LBG NQG GAEDG: YIGNV, DEEXG, YEUNTG. QLTMT BMT GE YBAZ QLNARG B YBA NG EAKZ FMTGGIMTJ NAQE KNXNAR EM JNGKNXNAR." — VMNGG WBYN, LTBKEKERZ

182. "U LWV TKL LK HKKG LKK NBW BXSBY. U QKFHY WSLUWS BO BT BTQXKW, JFL U OSS DVOSHN BO BHPBVO JSUTI JFOV, BTY U PBTL LXBL QKTTSQLUKT LK OAKWLO." – HUTYB QKXT

183. "U ZGLC FY FRUVH FRMF TYGUVS WMCL XYZ

WYOL RZVSOX MVC CLFLOWUVLC QZF MEFLO

WX GZJJLGG MF FRL YTXWIUJG MVC FRL Z.G.

YILV U OLMTUKL FRMF NUVVUVS UG FRL

QUSSLGF WYFUAMFUYV." -MVCX WZOOMX

184. "U'AP WPHGRUSCV QRZ NPHUJZB LQPS U

TPCG CUIP CUTP LRB LUSSUSM RSZ U LRB

CJBUSM, BJ U GQUSI PAPHVKJZV WRS

HPCRGP GJ GQRG YXRSZRHV — GQP

GPENGRGUJS GJ MUAP US, GJ MUAP XN, RSZ

GQPS LQRG UG GRIPB GJ IPPN MJUSM." -

ERCWJCE MPGB

185. "UFNV KQ S DEP VFN'U SCJSWY IN ANNG TSY,

SZY W'AA UFNV PNE S DEP PNE XSZ TQSI

QOQJP IWKQ." -ANE TJNXG

186. "U'J SHM T BUDJ IMTP, U TJ TS TQMPRII.

CRUSO T BUDJ IMTP UI IKQY T BTDIR DUBR,

DUERL BHP BTFR ETDKRI TSL BHP

GKCDUQUMX." — EUEURS DRUOY

187. "UL BFL IJMY IAJHH BI EFLBWI BFL WBEL ND,

BDE NJF GPAAGL GPHL PI FNJDELE UPAY B

IGLLQ." -UPGGPBW IYBOLIQLBFL, AYL

ALWQLIA

188. "ULKE GFEYKA YMFO'J MFYKKX GYEF LS

ULKE. JTFX'MF GYEF LS ADFYJ,

EFJFMGZOYJZLO, YOE Y TYME-JL-SZOE

YKKLX QYKKFE UWJA."– EYO UYNKF

189. "UNQGQ'P T UZCQ YNQK T CTK KQQXP UJ

LZWNU TKX T UZCQ YNQK NQ KQQXP UJ

TOOQHU UNTU NZP XQPUZKF'P DJPU, UNQ

PNZH NTP PTZDQX TKX UNTU JKDF T LJJD

YZDD OJKUZKAQ. UNQ UGAUN ZP Z'SQ

TDYTFP MQQK T LJJD." — IJNK TAWAPU

190. "UPB RFYGN XPN DL EDJL NP PBNNGFXM, PBN

RESMLN PS PBNQVLXZ UPBS HPRVLNFNFPX,

DBN UPB HEX PBNAPSM NGLR." – JPB GPJNT

191. "UYOM UYYJB XYA LTAP APM MVMB, EGA LTAP APM NTXZ, FXZ APMHMQYHM TB LTXI'Z SGRTZ RFTXAMZ EUTXZ." -LTUUTFN BPFJMBRMFHM, F NTZBGNNMH XTIPA'B ZHMFN

192. "V OEKU UCVMZ LVMMIGK LVM. BMR JENK LCH LHM BFF UCI LBN UCGHEJC CVJC KXCHHF BMR XHFFIJI, UCI TIKU QFBNIG BU IDIGN FIDIF, UCIN CBDI B LBN HS WBZVMJ UCVMJK CBQQIM BMR LVMMVMJ JBWIK." - UHMN REMJN

193. "VHBKR HLYM K ECRRMZVHU, NRLJS HLYM K EMM. RWM WKJXN OKJ'R WLR FWKR RWM MUMN OKJ'R NMM." – ICWKIIKX KHL

194. "VHN UY FH CYF FENHKCE FEY FHKCEYWF OYNJHSW JR UA GJVY, J EIS FH GHHT DJFEJR FH VJRS FEY YRYNCA FH SH JF. J SHR'F CJLY KO. RYLYN EILY. RYLYN DJGG." – BHRIE GHUK

195. "VIGL TMK CM FMZGRIWLU UMMC, RIG

JYUGLRWLG XGMXSG YGJSST JRRJNI

RIGZFGSHGF RM TMK. RIGT IJHG FM ZJLT

XYMQSGZF QJNE RIGYG RIJR RIGT'YG

SMMEWLU BMY FMZGQMCT RM QG XYMKC

MB. W RIWLE JQMKR RIJR, JLC W VML'R

BMYUGR WR." – ZJLK UWLMQWSW

196. "VKNAUYMD R QAABVRWWKL YE AMWX BPK QYLEB PRWQ AQ BPK EYWKMB GLRXKL R JYS AQQKLE OG BA BPK EJX AL NAMQYSKE BA PYE BKRNPKL YM R GLYURLX ENPAAW KEERX. BPK EKNAMS GRLB YE BPK MRUK AQ BPK BKRU PK TRMBE BA GWRX QAL." - RMSLKR GYLWA

197. "VP LVL MXP JTYP JXMK. VP VY XMJZ VM POR FXIVRY POTP DMVNR NVKOPRHY YPTU TML FVYY TML YJTYO TML FVYY TML PQYYJR XIRH YRIRHTJ SVPZ UJXSDY." — WTFRY WXMRY, NHXF ORHR PX RPRHMVPZ

198. "VRQ XIMEBMXJQ MY BGPXQVMEC LCLMEYV WGHIYQJD. MV'Y LNGHV YQJD-MPXIGKQPQEV, LNGHV NQMEC NQVVQI VRLE WGH UQIQ VRQ ZLW NQDGIQ." – YVQKQ WGHEC

199. "W UODN O AUNFQV AUOA PFDWNT FKNQOAN FI AUN YNDNY FG HQNOPT, MUNQN VFR HQNOP VFRQTNYG." — PNQVY TAQNNK

200. "WFPPYT SWI'U UZY WQVY QW LQPZ FT

LKGGZSWV. LKU SU SW FMUYI VFTY GYYJHD

MYHU UZQI TYHSASFI, QIG BKWU QW VKPZ Q

JQTU FM UZY PFVVKISUD'W MQLTSP, Q

TYJFWSUFTD FM UTQGSUSFIW." -MTQIEHSI

MFYT

201. "WG WPXFBPB TWGGKP VEG YCPX UKGBZ CG

XCI QKTHBPI. XB UEIP VEG YCPX XKQB CG

XCI XBWVP WGL LVBWUI CG XCI XBWL."–

BUCF SWPKQBH

202. "WJEBJD GTB LTKJRV KOMZDVVKBJV BY BQP OBCKD WILBZV KV YAJJE WUVBQALDQE IWJJBL UD LZAVLDP. K LTKJR KL'V QKRD W QWG BY JWLAZD." — VLDMTDJ RKJH, LTD GWVLD QWJPV

203. "WSFV LSDMY QDRKGYO LHV GYXYK HNDRW UHPFGC H KDVWYK DK NYFGC DG H WYHU. FW LHV HNDRW CFXFGC UOVYMI HG DBBDKWRGFWO. F LHGWYJ WD WHPY H KFVP, BRW UOVYMI DRW WSYKY HGJ BRW UO IHFWS FG HTWFDG. IHFWS LFWSDRW HTWFDG FV JYHJ. -QHKKOJ SHOGY

204. "WZMGO HLF HXUWDDX MT HLF UFWYMDWJQF ZMGNF...GH PGQQ RCWUWDHFF W NMESQWNFDNX MT DFZFU HUXGDR WDXHLGDR WOZFDHCUMCY..." — I. EGNLWFQ YHUWNAXDYBG

205. "X EAAO SAWZUM DVXMUT DVXMH YSUTU LSU DJWZ RH. X ETUXL SAWZUM DVXMUT DVXMH YSUTU LSU DJWZ RH EARKE LA QU." – YXMKU ETULHZM

206. "X IGA'W RPJA GA FYXAL IXDJRRGXAWYI. SY RPJA GA FYXAL QYJPPB LGGI, JAI GFEXGTDPB, SY RPJA GA SXAAXAL." – LQYLL WQGB

207. **"X'NN SG UWCEMJMB XE ECDMF EG UXP OCLMF, UWMEWMB XE'F FXEEXPO GP C RMPYW UCJXPO C EGUMN, WCPSXPO C YVA GQ UCEMB EG C EMCLLCEM, GB WXEEXPO EWM OCLM-UXPPXPO FWGE." -DGRM RBKCPE**

208. **"XETTANEEH'K KICHOE FMJ NJK GJMI EL J SETHFZ JSF UFDJCKF OI HOHZ'I ZFFH GMELJZOIA (CZTOWF MFJTOIA-IFTFPOKOEZ IEHJA)" — BJZZA GJDXFDE**

209. "XFGHPA IHUN HOUPSMPSHOL HO-YKIA KOR

WHRA KSP FMUPO ZSPAPOUPR KA QFXHQ,

UNP SHRHQDYP JSHOLHOL IPYQFXP SPYHPM

UF JPYPKLDPSPR XKSSHPR MFYWA

ADMMPSHOL FMMAQSPPO KU UNP NKORA FM

SPYKUHGPA." — EPKOHOP JKAHOLPS

210. "XLYLP RQPPG UTRLTXL JVT FTLUX'M ETYL

MVL RTYALU GTC ETYL. UTTXLP TP EQMLP,

MVQM ZLPUTX JAEE XTM ETYL GTC." — PTSLP

LDLPM

211. "XMK QSK XMGSC G RTGH TVV TVQSC GS XMK

NLGVH-LY (XQ CTPK XMJKK OMKS XMK TCKR

QA PTSZ PTJQQSR YVTZKJR OKJK MKTEGVZ

ILKRXGQSKH) GR ZQL DTSSQX NLZ

LSHKJRXTSHGSC. GX KGXMKJ KUGRXR QJ

GX HQKRS'X." – OTVVZ VKOGR

212. "XMMC KMGGYJ WAQFYJK UYYC UMB VY

BOBQUK KGTAWBYC VF POGNYAQUXYAM. OU

KMGGYJ, QVOAOBF OK PTGN PMJY

OPWMJBQUB BNQU KNQWY, QUC OU PQUF

GQKYK, KROAA OK BNY QJB MI BTJUOUX

AOPOBQBOMUK OUBM LOJBTYK." -YCTQJCM

XQAYQUM

213. "XRY PFFPHBCL CKCFXAWVHB PEERFLVHB AR

XRYF RZH APNAC, PHL NR V BRA AWC NPUC

APNACN PN XRY - RF CJNC V QFCACHLCL AR.

V PU FCPJJX HRA OYVAC NYFC ZWVEW - V

AWVHI NRUCAVUCN AWC RHC PHL

NRUCAVUCN AWC RAWCF." — WCHFVI VTNCH,

P LRJJ'N WRYNC

214. "XVA ISUZ'G IHHVJUM NIBF AZGEH XVA'QU

HUISZUM GV JEHHEZYHX TATOUZM

METNUHEUW." — SUNUBBI LASOPX,

OHABFEZY BAOEM'T NVJ

215. "Y HDBKM UVV WSH KKSL! UDE USSL! XGKT WSH IUVVHGM CSHD Y SYW TM EGYQHL. JRW Y'T IHWWYDI OGHWWM WYGHE KX WSH UCCL! UDE RSSL! CSHD Y TYLL U ORWW." – BKSD EUVM

216. "Y RLJM HCQM TUDTFU MD JUU VU CJ C XCIN-HDIGYQK EDDMSCFFUI CQN JDVUDQU HXD YJ TCJJYDQCMU CSDLM MXU KCVU." – NCBYN SUWGXCV

217. "Y XTQ MVJP XDOP DO LYQQOU ZO, Y UYOU XDOP DO EOCA ZO, Y EYIOU T COX XOOLQ XDYEO DO EVIOU ZO" — UVJVADR M DNWDOQ, YP T EVPOER SETBO

218. "YGDTFRDTY FNT FNROHY RO GLZ NTVXY VZT

QVZ CGZYT FNVO VOIFNROH FNTI WGLUX ALF

RO JGGMY GZ GO QRUD!!" — WM CTJJ

219. "YJ PKMMHJPP ZKH JTZFUZXP, JGUF ZKH

FNZKINFP, BXG DJNBAJ MZQUFJQS FZ FNJ

MZUXF ZL FJGUKT. XZ YZXGJH YJ PJJO

PZQBEJ UX FNJ JTZFUZXBQ BXG

MPSENZQZIUEBQ NZXJPFS ZL BX

KXLUQFJHJG TBOJ-DJQUJAJ YZHQG ZL

XZAJQP, TZAUJP, BXG MQBSP." — ONBXI

OUCBHHZ XIKSJX

220. "YLBYJL GROP PB YNBWLTP PZLCN BGO

COXLTDNCPCLX BO BPZLNX, HDP C NLVDXL

PB RJJBG PZLU PB YDP PZRP BO UL. WDXP

HLTRDXL QBD SBO'P PZCOA PZRP QBD TBDJS

HL PZL HLXP CO PZL GBNJS SBLXO'P ULRO

PZRP C XZBDJSO'P ZRFL PZL TBOVCSLOTL PB

HLJCLFL C TRO SB ROQPZCOI." —NBOSR

NBDXLQ

221. "YLH APSCY YLUIK TOPJY XPNUH-XTGUIK UC

YLTY UY'C QUGH QUBH: IPOPEF VTI KP OTVG

YP VPSSHVY YLH XUCYTGHC." — MTJQUIH

GTHQ, GUCC GUCC OTIK OTIK: BUQX

ASUYUIKC, 1965-1967

222. "YM NSHPP SWP WLC THIWDYGLPSYA DG MYIK-KWEYLQ, YD UGJIF XH YL DSH UWC YD SHIAP CGJ FHOHIGA AWDYHLNH WLF FYPNYAIYLH YL NSGGPYLQ XHDUHHL WIDHTLWDYOHP WD W DYKH USHL WL YKAJIPYOH FHNYPYGL PHHKP OHTC WDDTWNDYOH." — PDWLIHC EJXTYNE

223. "YNI CY GIWPCSA NIP HOWDM TPIYY. YNI CYS'R DPLCSA, HZR YNI SIBIP TCT DPL, WSLNJG. CR'Y W HPCANR YZSSL TWL WST YNI'Y OCMI W HOWDM YNWTJG DPIIQCSA TJGS RNI IEQRL YRPIIR." — VIWS-QWZO YWPRPI, SJ IUCR WST RNPII JRNIP QOWLY

224. "YO YMPKL MQMT SAG BGKKHSJ YS RMOK

QRMYKOKG YRSAZRYL QK QMVY. LS HS

URSYSZGMURL, JSOXKL, MVH YRK

XVYKGVKY. YRKT UGSOXHK AL QXYR JSGK

XVYKFFKNYAMF LYXJAFX, CAY YRKT

NSVLYGANY M FSQKG, RMGHKG NKXFXVZ." —

NRANP PFSLYKGJMV

225. "YRQP HP YRQ TLGHPC TIVQYRHPC

RKLLQPQB YI VQ. XQT, H GQVQVSQG. H DQJJ

HP JIUQ FHYR EKVQT YXGIPQ KPB FKT TI

RKLLX DIG YHVQ." — QMCQPQ I'PQHJJ, JIPC

BKX'T EIMGPQX HPYI PHCRY

226. "YS AQJGWOL QDRQSL OTDZ YG OT NG OBG

LQYG AGJLTW WT YQOOGJ KE STH'JG WT.1

KW OBG RTJDZ TJ WT. 1000. KO ZTGLW'O

YQOOGJ. QDRQSL NG ATDKOG QWZ QDRQSL

NG JGLAGMOEHD OTRQJZL TOBGJL." –

MQJTDKWG RTXWKQMFK

227. "YWXXDOSU UQCL DWM SWYRQXQ. OG DWM

CMXS MV YWXXDOSU KPWMC RWY DWM'XQ

UWOSU CW VQXGWXZ, DWM'NQ KBXQKJD

BWLC. CXKOS RKXJ, CMXS MV, XMS DWMX

PQLC KSJ CRQ XQLC YOBB CKIQ EKXQ WG

OCLQBG." – MLKOS PWBC

228. "YZ Y BWNDP YPR OKDDKDP KF DWZ ZGR

EWFZ KETWCZYDZ ZGKDP... ZGR KETWCZYDZ

ZGKDP KF ZW QRJRUWT VCRYZKJR YDQ

FLKUURQ TUYBRCF OKZG PWWQ

VWDHKQRDVR." -YCFRDR ORDPRC

229. "YZIUI RUI FHUI YZTCPE TC ZIRMIC RCX

IRUYZ, ZHURYTH, YZRC RUI XUIRFY HK TC

BHSU LZTAHEHLZB." - GTAATRF EZRJIELIRUI,

ZRFAIY

230. "YZZ UQK GYJ BQ TA IW UQKS IWAX AWZN.

T'L SWMSWAWJXTJH LQSW XFYJ DKAX LW. T

XFTJV WRWSU MWSAQJ AFQKZB XFTJV XFYX

CYU." – LTAXU GQMWZYJB

231. "Z IKUMZUXPV MK IBNN PYPOF SPPD XUMZN

Z EZUBNNF IBXRJM JZG. Z MJZUD ZM'W

WBEP MK WBF MJBM MJZW ZW SJPOP Z

HPRBU MK NPBOU MJBM QPOWZWMPUIP

QBFW KEE." – LXWMZU OKHPOMW ZU HPWM

WPBM ZU MJP JKXWP

232. "ZAK QGWGO OGJPPZ KQRGOCYJQR J

VGOCAQ KQYLP ZAK DAQCLRGO YELQXC

SOAF ELC VALQY AS WLGH ... KQYLP ZAK

DPLFT LQCLRG AS ELC CULQ JQR HJPU

JOAKQR LQ LY." -EJOVGO PGG, YA ULPP J

FADULQXTLOR

233. "ZAPPFB QKFBBZVC [AC LGK DGACK,

HFBMXBBFCJ MVBLFCJ YAP GFB ZAUFK]:

"QGVL VSAXL MEVXHKLLK MAESKPL? BGK'B

SPFLFBG, FBC'L BGK? BGK BAXCHB SPFLFBG.

FB BGK, EFNK, VYYKMLKH AP FB BGK

SPFLFBG?" — OXEFVC YKEEAQKB, JABYAPH

DVPN: LGK BGAALFCJ BMPFDL

234. "ZAQP ZAWK AKPIW, LAC BDAE, IPWN KPAKNP

KIPJPDMHDX JA GP TWBP KPAKNP EHJF

QWMP-CK KIAGNPQZ GPHDX EWJRFPM GL

IPWN KPAKNP JA TAIXPJ JFPHI IPWN

KIAGNPQZ." — RFCRB KWNWFDHCB, RFABP

235. "ZJSY XY XYIGE VXIV RZZLQ IGY IBMIAQ RYVVYG VXIJ PZHKYQ, ROV XY JZM LJYM VXIV PZHKYQ IGY RYVVYG VXIJ VXY GYIB BKCY." — EIHZG RIJZHKS, WKGB MKVX RGZLYJ OPRGYBBI

236. "ZJX HXTA CJA QRQN TAJI DQGCM FPGHTGOUW. UCV ZJX HXTA CJA, QRQN, MGRQ UCZJCQ QWTQ APQ NQTIJCTGDGWGAZ KJN ZJXN WGKQ." — HUNZ JWGRQN, FGWV MQQTQ

237. "ZPEQPWTL CWPS E VEQPO ZUHTH XMQ 600

UEZP ETJ HTJ BV ZWTLWTL MT PMV MX E

LWETP HGHVSETP...JMHZ WP LHP ETO

IHPPHQ PSET PSWZ?" — HCET KULQHLMQ

238. "ZROIO'P YG HWVUQWIN WYN YG JGIQWIN, YG

NWE GZROI ZRWY ZRBP. EGT JBFF EGTI VWIZ

WP EGT KG, WYN ZRWZ'P ZRWZ." — DGRY

HTIYRWS PVRQWIZA, YGIZRQOPZ VGIYOI

239. "ZVTE QHY YXT LHJT KVRE 3-5% HO QHYJ

MJRBE, QHY GHE'K ZREK KH MT HE TRJKV!" -

MHM GBRLHEG, BEKTJGBLTEXBHERI

RKKHJETQ, OJHL KVT RIMTJK MJHHPX'

LHDBT, GTOTEGBEA QHYJ IBOT"

240. "DUXJNARMVRD VZ X RUIYXJ SUP, ZCIA. LUK KUCJM QUC JVFA VN VR QUCI SUP VT ABAIQ NVYA QUC YXMA X ZYXJJ YVZNXFA, X IAM JVDLN KARN UR UBAI QUCI MAZF XRM 15,000 HAUHJA ZNUUM CH XRM QAJJAM XN QUC?" - SXWOCAZ HJXRNA

241. A'T RGJYARO, ATWIBAGPB IPV I JABBJG APRGXFCG. A TIUG TARBIUGR, A IT ZFB ZY XZPBCZJ IPV IB BATGR OICV BZ OIPVJG. NFB AY MZF XIP'B OIPVJG TG IB TM LZCRB, BOGP MZF RFCG IR OGJJ VZP'B VGRGCQG TG IB TM NGRB. -TICAJMP TZPCZG

242. ABH SVMN FB GNDENTF QWI QIKVGN

DBKNBWN UCBK ABH SBON, PHF QTFHQSSA,

ABH SBON NONW KBGN FCN ENBESN UCB

GNYHVGN HWINGDFQWIVWJ QWI UCB KQMN

KVDFQMND QWI CQON FB JGBU UVFC FCNVG

KVDFQMND. -NSNQWBG GBBDNONSF

243. ACY JYOKZJ AH XY GHRYJ BE ACY PLYKAYEA

HN KGG KLLHPKZA WLYESOWABHZE. -

NLBYJLBTC ZBYAMETCY

244. AD AH QKX YRQAYNH DRGD HRQZ ZRGD ZN

DXKTP GXN, JGX WQXN DRGS QKX

GMATADANH.- F.L. XQZTASE, RGXXP CQDDNX

GSI DRN YRGWMNX QJ HNYXNDH

245. **AFEHB IWCPM DEFPUPUX CAAIC DT CGFRA DGA BTWUX JEFPU, CDEAUXDGAUPUX DGA UAWEFH MTUUAMDPTUC FUQ RAEGFRC ACDFJHPCGPUX UAK TUAC. -QE. SEFUMAC EFWCMGAE**

246. **AGQRE RQ QSAWZVROJ ZVKZ QVSGYB QLWKT MSC RZQWYM, QZCKRJVZ MCSA ZVW VWKCZ. RZ ZSST AW K YSOJ ZRAW ZS GOBWCQZKOB ZVKZ. -BKASO KYPKCO**

247. **AHBT PO ZN FTAPCPHV — P EHJAY YPT SHF IQWI — P EHJAY YPT SHF NHJ. ZN EFTTY PO AHBT WVY NHJ WFT PIO HVAN ITVTI. -DHQV GTWIO**

248. AJWFN FW I ATMIG GIP. FE DFOUW WTJG ET EYU JCFOUMWU, PFCDW ET EYU AFCQ, XGFDYE ET EYU FAIDFCIEFTC, ICQ NYIMA ICQ DIFUEZ ET GFXU ICQ ET UOUMZEYFCD. -RGIET

249. AML XYACPTAL YLKKHO TYY HS XK MTQL AH YLTVO CK XORHOGCACHOTY YHQL, UMCRM CORYXGLK OHA HOYI HAMLVK NXA HXVKLYQLK TK ULYY. -LYCBTNLAM DXNYLV-VHKK

250. ANVLW? ANVLW LV YLBH! LX'V IMZVLWRY

HAEXLEQ - ZEN WRQ XENWM LX! LX'V QHEQ

HWXE-HQHKFZ VNWSHG ENX EB VILKLXV

RQG VCLXWMHG LQXE VENQG CRTHV BEK

ZENK HRKV XE VCRYYEC. RKH ZEN XHYYLQF

AH, CMRX, XMRX LX'V DEKLQF? ZEN GEQ'X

MRTH XLAH BEK LX? — LVRRW ARKLEQ

251. APSABO OPDZ JCKM...JCKM CO XMDX DO PSIF

DO CJ CO UMCIF APCABMX SWW UZ PCJJPM

YGMMPO; SIPZ YGMI JGM APSAB OJSRO

XSMO JCKM ASKM JS PCWM. -YCPPCDK

WDQPBIMT, JGM OSQIX DIX JGM WQTZ

252. APT LPE'F UPKR ZPDRPER SPN FJRMN UPPIZ,

PN FJRMN HUPFJRZ, PN SPN FJRMN SVEHA

HVN, CTF CRHVTZR FJRA ZMEO V ZPEO PEUA

APT HVE JRVN. -PZHVN XMULR

253. ATTQ YMDT LU ZMHW ITXWJ. X YLRT ELJIMHJ

LJ LG YLAT X GHUYTGG CXWSTU EITU JIT

RYMETWG XWT STXS. JIT FMUGFLMHGUTGG

MR YMDLUC XUS KTLUC YMDTS KWLUCG X

EXWBJI XUS WLFIUTGG JM YLRT JIXJ

UMJILUC TYGT FXU KWLUC. -MGFXW ELYST

254. AUR QNK'S QUIA NKAXUCA NKC ZKC LVSB NKASBVKM. VG AUR QUIA, VS PZNKE AUR'DZ LUDHVKM LVSBURS NKA DZNJ GZZJVKM. KU SLU IZUIJZ UK ZNDSB NDZ NJVHZ, NKC VS'E MUS SU XZ SBNS LNA VK PREVQ UD VS VEK'S PREVQ. — XVJJVZ BUJVCNA

255. AZEH PL KZWH QDVI BMLQ V UHHAPIN: PQ'L V GWZSHLL WHRMPWPIN SZIQPIMVA VQQHIQPZI. AZEPIN THAA QVJHL AVMNDQHW, AZOVAQO, VIF TVIQPIN KZWH QZ CH VCAH QZ LVO, 'P MIFHWLQVVIF' QDVI QZ DHVW, 'OZM'WH WPNDQ.' -KZAAHHI KVQLMKMWV

256. B LKOO KO B FHCWFX QYKUL VWOKJMWV PX

MBQTYW QH OQHG OGWWUA DAWM DHYVO

PWUHRW OTGWYSFTHTO. -KMJYKV PWYJRBM

257. B YPKQW B SJRTML'I TJUK ZJR HJWK IDQL B

MJ WBADI LJP, QLM ZKI B OLJP B PBTT

IJHJWWJP. -TKJ SDWBYIJCDKW

258. B'X ECKPI HBTM BAWVMO HNKX CMBAU EA

KPIOIEARBAU UKGHMN. IVEI'O IVM

RBOIEAWM XD GMHI MEN BO HNKX XD NBUVI.

-CMA WNMAOVEJ

259. BC GUBHQ OH UQTIOHBOV IUOHY B GURBUWU BH NLOX B AT OHA BH IJ ODX TD IMYBV, XLUH BH XLOX DUYSUVX JTM VOH VORR IU XLOX... B GURBUWU BH NLOX B AT, OHA B'RR YOJ BX. -FTLH RUHHTH

260. BCKY, OPEQ OQ PJ GJAZKSOQJZ CR TCSK WQPMQ; ILQKQ ZLQKQ GA LPZKQY, BQZ OQ ACI BCXQ; ILQKQ ZLQKQ GA GJVSKT, WPKYCJ; ILQKQ ZLQKQ GA YCSHZ, RPGZL; ILQKQ ZLQKQ GA YQAWPGK, LCWQ; ILQKQ ZLQKQ GA YPKEJQAA, BGDLZ; PJY ILQKQ ZLQKQ GA APYJQAA, VCT. -RKPJMGA CR PAAGAG

261. BCWMTPCL KJGMT EWPCL NJG PZ

AQGMBPCUW KJGMT UPSPCL NJG. – RJZQHT

TQUUQG, ABMAT-22

262. BEPA UCC NZFJ HPIKJPI UJP HKIOKCCPH, NZF

BKCC GUIO MFIO OBZ SZOPI: OZ CZSP DZJP,

UAH LP EUXXN. -EURKY ZR XPJIKU

263. BFKM WFNAIMBE EVAIS JTC MKMAWSRVTX

MBIM EJBBI VTSF BVTM. WFN AMJBBW RJKM

SF BFKM WFNAIMBE SF XMS JTWSRVTX CFTM

VT SRVI ZFABC. -BNGVBBM PJBB

264. BGDY REP'WD OY UEFD, OX'J XGD CEJX

TUEWOEPJ XBE-VYK-V-GVUL KVRJ EL REPW

UOLD. -WONGVWK UDBOJ

265. BIBYL OEUKP OEDO LGJ QGIB, LGJ NUQQ

BIBKOJDQQL QGXB, WJO UK OEB BKZ, QGIB

NUQQ YBOJYK UK D ZUHHBYBKO HGYV. -

HYDKR TDHTD

266. BK B FXT SYPN X IBJ JBMFAOYC X PBIBTU AC

YOYT X NXMMBAT KAC DQMBF BT LSYBC

PBKY, LSYT LSXL'M X VATJYCKQP LSBTU. -

YJJBY OXT SXPYT

267. BL YMCTBIF, BL TGZM INMYM BH C

RMYVCLMLI HSEEMYBLQ UNBDN PGF

LMSIYCTBWMH, YMLKMYH ZBYISCT, KMTCFH,

XSI UNBDN DCL CI CLF VGVMLI XMDGVM UNCI

BI UGSTK NCZM XMDGVM TGLQ MCYTBMY BE

GLM NCK LGI GXICBLMK UNCI GLM UCLIMK,

CIYGDBGSH. -VCYDMT RYGSHI

268. BLNAWLX P VIHAS MLUXLL IH NBALVVNULBDL

BIX NCPUNBPANIB BIX RIAW AIULAWLX UI AI

AWL CPFNBU IH ULBNZG. VIOL, VIOL, VIOL,

AWPA NG AWL GIZV IH ULBNZG. -JIVHUPBU

PCPMLZG CIYPXA

269. **BMQZ LP OFZ QLXOSZ MK OFZ FZHXO,**

PLGNZXLOJ LP OFZ QLXOSZ MK OFZ ELGW,

WZNLPLMG LP OFZ QLXOSZ MK OFZ TLBB,

NMSXHRZ LP OFZ QLXOSZ MK OFZ PCLXLO. -

KXHGI BBMJW TXLRFO

270. **BPIY HIQAM I XCCW ECCQ IOW BPIY HIQAM I**

XCCW HCKSA ILA YCYIVVZ WSJJALAOY

YPSOXM. –MAYP XLIPIHA-MHSYP

271. BS FUWQ UR BDUO PSIFM ZSG EGOB JQ TJFQ

BS MS BDIQQ BDURHO: BS FSWQ PDTB UO

ESIBTF; BS DSFM UB THTUROB ZSGI JSRQO

VRSPURH ZSGI SPR FUCQ MQKQRMO SR UB;

TRM, PDQR BDQ BUEQ YSEQO BS FQB UB HS,

BS FQB UB HS. -ETIZ SFUWQI

272. BSDP ODUK QAIEP – PSK UYEAO VI PSK

UAEKIF? CAC A RAEPKH PV PSK UYEAO

JKODYEK A BDE UAEKIDJRK? VI BDE A

UAEKIDJRK JKODYEK A RAEPKHKC PV PSK

UYEAO? CV DRR PSVEK IKOVICE PYIH FVY

AHPV D UKRDHOSVRF LKIEVH? — HAON

SVIHJF, SAWS QACKRAPF

273. **BSDYW'E YWB DAHWY IGSTB JLD GLKB. A**

NLX'Y ZXLP PWBDB AY'E GAZBGU YL HL

OBYYBD. -DLOBDY JDLEY

274. **BSKL MD YPL DYEXIVL ZLNMBULECLIY NPMJP**

SKLEYXTLD SIL GLEDSI SI XJJSQIY SR

XISYPLE GLEDSI. -FXCLD YPQEZLE

275. **BTS HJS BTUJI PS YNJ JSGSK ISB SJHRIT HL**

UE XHGS. NJW BTS HJS BTUJI PS YNJ JSGSK

IUGS SJHRIT HL UE XHGS. -TSJKA CUXXSK

276. BXUF AJOK YKOYI. FWHKFCC AJOK BJUF.

CIZKF AJOK FMYIOCXZCS. YZEF ZDYXJM

YJQZKTC AJOK TKFZSC. QZBE AJOK YZBE.

TZMDF ZMT CXMR YJ AJOK SOCXD. FSNKZDF

AJOK NBFCCXMRC. SZEF YJTZA QJKYI

KFSFSNFKXMR. -CYFUF SZKZNJBX

277. BYL: O KC K JUYKCYU. WGU K JUYKCYU OL

GAY REG DKA GAMB WOAJ EOL RKB NB

CGGAMOVEF, KAJ EOL XSAOLECYAF OL FEKF

EY LYYL FEY JKRA NYWGUY FEY UYLF GW

FEY RGUMJ. – GLDKU ROMJY, FEY DUOFOD KL

KUFOLF

278. BYTQ EQMZN VMTWZJ FY NMI IYC'PQ NYPPI

QTQPI RWRFQQZ EWZCFQN. -GYVZ BQZZYZ

279. C PWEF DAF NFPJDCWSMACV DAJD JSBWSF

AJM QCDA GOMCK ... RFKJOMF DAFNF'M

MWGFDACSH CS OM DAJD CM RFBWSL DAF

NFJKA WU QWNLM, MWGFDACSH DAJD

FPOLFM JSL LFUCFM WON RFMD JDDFGVDM

DW MVCD CD WOD. ... CD'M DAF RFMD VJND

WU OM VNWRJRPB ... — SCKT AWNSRB,

280. C WVAX MERJQ IWX HVFVQEP, IWVI CM OER

NEAX RJICN CI WRFIK, IWXFX BVJ GX JE

YEFX WRFI, EJNO YEFX NEAX. -YEIWXF

IXFXKV

281. CAE BOG QIVGOPGSJ, CAE BOG MQOGL PAO KJOEXXTG, WEJ CAE BOG MAOJRC AP TAHG BFL WGTAFXQFX. -WOGFG WOAMF

282. CAUQ AB OLVQ OF QVJF VU SFTDI TCKAEQVDQ TU DAQ CVQFETVH, OLFQLFE TQ'U CMUTX AE BFFHTDIU AE HAWF. QLFG'EF QLTDIU OF XVD'Q EFVHHG UFF AE QAMXL. QLFG'EF DAQ CVQFETVH, SMQ QLFG'EF WTQVHHG TCKAEQVDQ QA MU. -RMZG XAHHTDU

283. **CB ERNQCOV, QUZR CI NGUAO GRLUDCBF OXR**

ECFXO HREIUB. WUB'O QUUP TUE OXR

HREIUB VUA MNBO OU IHRBW VUAE QCTR

MCOX. GRLUDR OXR HREIUB VUA MNBO OU

IHRBW VUAE QCTR MCOX. -BRCQ IOENAII

284. **CJNSXJUW COHU IJ NS, 'XAI IGS XSOIDSC**

TSQS OMIH-NOISQHODHCIHL.' IGOI'C O GAPS

NWIG. RJGM OMU H DHISQODDW ACSU IJ CHI

UJTM OMU COW, 'MJT, DSI'C TQHIS O

CTHNNHMP EJJD. — EOAD NLLOQIMSW

285. CJZR XP GNXRBKPUXI OUWO UWP MWQVUO

GXNR. XO XP SQXRO QBKRNPOWBKXBV,

EQOQWC MJBGXKRBMR, PUWNXBV WBK

GJNVXZXBV. XO XP CJAWCOA OUNJQVU

VJJK WBK HWK OXERP. XO PROOCRP GJN

CRPP OUWB IRNGRMOXJB WBK EWLRP

WCCJFWBMRP GJN UQEWB FRWLBRPPRP. -

WBB CWBKRNP

286. CUD YVKD OGK FEE NEEZ FSB AKGSHZ, CUD

YFKDZ, CUD ZGKKGAZ FSB CUD YKNJDZ GO

UVJFSNCT, FEE END NS CUD GSD AGKB

'EGPD.' NC NZ CUD BNPNSD PNCFENCT CUFC

DPDKTAUDKD RKGBVYDZ FSB KDZCGKDZ

ENOD. -ETBNF JFKNF YUNEB

287. D KIWP, DS RIIJXQCIP XWT RIIP FDUUIT DP W

YUWPI HOWNX WJ JBIPJZ-JBQ, JXI XDNJQOZ

QS KENDH BQEUT XWCI RIIP CIOZ TDSSIOIPJ.

WN BQEUT JXI XDNJQOZ QS WCDWJDQP, QS

HQEONI. — JQK NJQYYWOT, JXI OIWU JXDPM

288. D XLWI UILUXI. D XLWI BZ MQBDXZ, BZ

HYDXROIG... FTV DGJDRI BZJIXM DJ Q UXQHI

EYIOI D XDWI QXX QXLGI QGR VYQV'J EYIOI

ZLT OIGIE ZLTO JUODGNJ VYQV GIWIO ROZ

TU. -UIQOX J. FTHP

289. DCYM FBP'HY UVINMS V UBZNY BQ V GBBI,

XYBXEY VHY VEDVFL DVNANMS DNAC ACYNH

IMNZYL. –RBYE YTSYHABM

290. DEW VAELG ED XEZ CP VAG KAGYN LGYVL, C'T

RCHG XY VE KRYN XEZW AYPTL VE VACL

EPG; VAG WGLV ED XEZ KYP UZLV WYVVRG

XEZW UGJGRWX! — UEAP RGPPEP

291. DM ZY ZFDI ESIDN ZY'VY VYFKA, ZY'NN GY

ZFDIDSO MLV IBY VYRI LM LEV NDUYR. –

NYHLSA RSDWXYI, IBY YVRFIC YNYUFILV

292. DO VHO VWW FK LCO QTLLOH, GTL EPSO PM

TE VHO WPPIFKQ VL LCO ELVHE. – PEJVH

DFWXO, WVXU DFKXOHSOHO'E MVK

293. DSLHU HLC'V PSLV J YKGJLSNG, J

VNJCLHGCV LJVHLBJUVHFC. HV'L J CGGM, J

MGGY WSCOGN; JCM ZWGC VWG DSLHU HL

NHOWV, HV'L PFR. KFEG. J BFNGVJLVG FB

WGJEGC. -FNLFC LUFVV UJNM

294. DU'W LT EWV QTDLQ FIMS UT CVWUVPJIC,

FVMIEWV D OIW I JDYYVPVLU AVPWTL UBVL.

– HVODW MIPPTHH, IHDMV'W IJGVLUEPVW DL

OTLJVPHILJ

295. DW HTD, BWV TDU JWDZMQKVTXPK GKVMWQ,

JTD AKTV WDK BTJK LW EMHZKPB TDQ

TDWLEKV LW LEK HSPLMLSQK, AMLEWSL

BMDTPPU FKLLMDF XKAMPQKVKQ TZ LW

AEMJE HTU XK LEK LVSK. - DTLETDMKP

ETALEWVDK, LEK ZJTVPKL PKLLKV

296. DZUG ZK IGPXZXTDGKK QXDW ZU VG PDDQV ZH HQ EG. GPSL QU NK LPK HLG BQVGM HQ TZJG DZUG IGPXZXT, HQ IPFG QNM HZIG PXC QNM EQCZGK PXC QNM VQMCK ZXHQ ZXKHMNIGXHK QU DQJG PXC LQBG. -HQI LGPC

297. E CMHEMQM AGPA P NMTZRU'Z APZAM EU KJZEW AMHHZ XRJ P HRA PCRJA AGMK. EU ZRKM WPZMZ, EA AMHHZ XRJ MQMTXAGEUD XRJ UMML AR IURO. — HMEHP ZPHMZ, AGEZ ZRUD OEHH ZPQM XRJT HEVM

298. E VQLNH SOON VUIV VUOQO IQO ID WIBH ZIHD

RS NRAEBJ ID VUOQO IQO KORKNO EB VUO

ZRQNF IBF ID VUOQO IQO FIHD EB VUO NESO

RS VURDO KORKNO. -WIQH D. MINFOQRBO

299. E WFR'N CRFJ (EV NQKI JKMK PKR FM JFPKR

VYRG MXRRERH RYCKW YLMFGG NQK

VEKUW). NQKI QYW TYHG FZKM NQKEM

QKYWG. -IFHE TKMMY

300. EC EL EYOVNS, BNY TEL'O XMQXTO E ANRHX

ON DX EL HFFYCOSEOHNL NK OVX DNNP. HK

OVEO'C JVEO BNY VNQX KNS, BNY

CVNYFUL'O CXFF OVX SHIVOC. –DXSLVESU

CTVFHLP

301. EDKL CLSDNMQILA MD RYCCQLCA. QH UFVJA

BFCXELA, ELYJA WLMSLA, JLMLHCYHLA

GYEEA HD YCCQKL YH QHA XLAHQMYHQDM

WFEE DW BDJL. -VYTY YMNLEDF

302. EFAK DQW NBA RHNCRKRKC, DQW HRCFZ NG

EAII RHNCRKA GQHAZFRKC EQBZFEFRIA. –

IWJD HNWL HQKZCQHABD, NKKA QO CBAAK

CNVIAG

303. EFFGWSUFX GFTTC OSJ DWPG VG'C TVLF GS

EF EFFGWSUFX PXB QSYPIG GFTTC OSJ DWPG

VG'C TVLF GS EF WJQPX. EPRW GFTTC OSJ

DWPG VG'C TVLF GS EF GWF JXVUFICF. -

BSJMTPC PBPQC

304. EG USIJ LFCIOE SMR TGEECKDR HYEL SE DGIO

SE JGY BGI'L PIGN LFRJ'MR CUTGEECKDR. –

IGMLGI HYELRM, LFR TFSILGU LGDDKGGLF

305. EJOUW UO D NDBHRN PUFHR NI EH MX PIY. D

EHYUJE DRY D CBDNGIKE DRY D SDX NI

OCKHDY D EHOODPH IG KUPTNHIJORHOO... D

EHOODPH IG BIFH, D EHOODPH IG JRUNX. -

ONHCTHR EDKBHX

306. EL DPX EPMW WK VKGL KWRLS QLKQVL

EFWRKCW RKVUFMY OPAZ, WK ILLV

PCWRLMWFA, WK OSLPWRL FM WRL OLPCWX

PSKCMU CT, WK UPMAL PMU TFMY. XLW LPAR

UPX EL VFTWLM WK FMMLS GKFALT WRPW

ZLLQ KCS VFIL TDPVV. -WPSP OSPAR

307. E'P CGIK IVB JH OB TKEAIXG IXXEKG HJK XSG

CJKMP XJ FGG. NDX E CJDMP KIXSGK SIAG IV

JTGV HMGFS CJDVP XSIV GAGK CGIK I NIVP-

IEP EV TDNMEZ. — MIPB WIWI

308. EPMXM OY GIEPOGL TIXM EI UM YNOJ IX EI

UM JIGM EIGOLPE, YI PNGJ TM IFMX TK

FOISOG NGJ SME CY EXK EI DIXLME DIX PNSD

NG PICX EPM TOYMXNUSM QMNEPMX NGJ

EPM YEOSS TIXM TOYMXNUSM QNKY ID ICX

DMSSIQTMG. -NXEPCX RIGNG JIKSM

309. EPVFEZ ZVMLG BLNR FNP ZNY PTCC OV RNLV

QTGMHHNTFEVQ OZ EJV EJTFWG EJME ZNY

QTQF'E QN EJMF OZ EJV NFVG ZNY QTQ QN. –

J.XMUSGNF OLNPF XL., H.G. T CNIV ZNY

310. EQPF P QPHHB PMR QTDB OPCQZTM ZF ZC

FQPF FQTCA EQT DTYA TMA PMTFQAS

CQTXDR SACF TM FQA CPWA HZDDTE. -

MPFQPMZAD QPEFQTSMA

311. ERNS FU VGS OTUKSJ, DHV KGFES XRH OJS

KOFVFTZ PRJ VGS OTUKSJ USQ JOFUSU URIS

AJSVVX ZRRB MHSUVFRTU. -KRRBX OEEST

312. EWDPD HJ WBPFZL B IMPD XPBRHMOJ XHQE

EWBE YD RBU MQQDP JMIDKMFL EWBU EM

BRRDNE EWDI QOZZL, EM ZMCD EWDI BZIMJE

FDJNHED EWDIJDZCDJ. -DZHGBKDEW

XHZKDPE

313. EWHNVKMV NY HFV QWGX ZJ HGLV DZUV. NJ TZL HGLDT DZUV YZQVZKV, TZL BNDD CV QZGV EWHNVKH BNHF HFWH EVGYZK. - HFNMF KFWH FWKF

314. EWVQX XDPYTVPV HIP WTUPCVHYTUQTJ; QTVGQCPV QH, YTU DQAHV QH QTHL Y CPYDE ZIQXI QH ZLWDU TLH CPYXI QA QH ZPCP DPAH HL QHVPDA. -IPTCB ZYCU MPPXIPC

315. EWZUK NLWKPFUCY ZFUEWAPFNZ,

KOPAANYSNZ, PYL NYMUKONZ CWM GCWYS

DNCDAN LWMUYS FONUM XCMEPFUBN,

ZKOCCA GNPMZ; UFZ BPAWN APZFZ P

AUXNFUEN. -FPEEG VPALQUY

316. EY TYC PGYM LBYLKB MQY AGDADX XQBT

KAPB 'OKK PAGED YV ICDAF'. XQOX

OFXCOKKT IBOGD XQBT KAPB GY PAGED YV

ICDAF. -FQCFP PKYDXBNIOG

317. F MVD VB HNXQ HV, 'YWX, XVH, QFX F XVHA-AQU.' A DWMM 'WU, 'A TVE'D REVG FEX.' DYWX GFED UW DV UFRW VEW NS. A TVE'D UFRW 'WU NS. A TVE'D WOWE REVG GYWE A QFX AD. DYWX'IW DYW DINDY. FET AD AQ DYW DINDY. A TVE'D REVG. -XVHA LWIIF

318. FAXJITK JWWEPTDJEW JX HAKK EH YTWNUS DE DZU XDTDU, HES CZUW FEYUX EH FAXJI IZTWNU, DZU HAWYTFUWDTK KTCX EH DZU XDTDU TKCTBX IZTWNU CJDZ DZUF. -QKTDE

319. FBQP ZE Y VYUP JCYJ JXB NYK SFYD YKH LBJC XZK. -PQY VYLBO

320. FBUUFW FWEQZW HENWHEFF BN E AWYX

QJJR UGBVQ HWPEZNW BU MWWON UGW

OEYWVUN JII UGW NUYWWUN. -XJQB HWYYE

321. FCSWXRS DRMCB SX OVBXNKSV CS, SCDV CM

PRMS K GRQBW XJ GXNCQL INXORBSCXQ

OVKOZCQVM XN OKSVM GT FWCBW GCZZM

DRMS GV IKCO. -JNKQU EKIIK

322. FELYD YL OIZ MNZBO EWYOZN. BW

YWDNZXYGPZ QHNDZ. LHFZOIYWM OIBO

TZHTPZ RIH XYQQZN HW ZJZNAOIYWM BWX

BWAOIYWM ZPLZ DBW IBJZ YW DHFFHW. -

LBNBI XZLLZW

323. FG ZAW BMUO'C VAAL BC YAEFOV

ZAWMQUYG, ZAW PFYY NBEU B LFGGFXWYC

CFJU YAEFOV BOZAOU, QFOXU ZAW'YY

MUQUOC CNU CFJU BOL UOUMVZ ZAW VFEU

BOACNUM KUMQAO CNBC ZAW BMUO'C UEUO

VFEFOV CA ZAWMQUYG. -HBMHBMB LU

BOVUYFQ

324. F'L QRWXQUZ PWQAZ. F'L Q NXQWRXEE

MXWESC. F IGFCY FI PWXXME VM SC ZSV. F

USC'I IGFCY FI PQC OX EISMMXU. FN LZ

UXEIFCZ FE IS RSEX LZ LFCU OXPQVEX SN

NQLX, IGXC IGQI'E LZ UXEIFCZ. OVI LZ

MQEEFSC EIFRR LXQCE LSWX IGQC

QCZIGFCH. — RQUZ HQHQ

325. FLAQPLYB INFU EHOQ AQ H FWLSQV VHYXL.

UWHMRF H TLU. YL BLN VQHTTB SHMU

ANFXG XM UWQ FWLSQV? X ENQFF UWQVQ'F

ML PQUUQV CTHGQ UL YHMGQ UWHM H

FTXGR FNVZHGQ MQKU UL H ETHFF YLLV. —

IQVVB FQXMZQTY

326. FLYK JD VUK QULFK UJDVLCA LN P QLZPG'D

FJNK, JV JD XEV PG KRJDLBK JG P ZPG'D. -

ZPBPZK BK DVPKF

327. FMTI RVMIA MJQ VYLQ CVMTL KEQKLA. DEQ

MKDSJA MTH HYJQKDSJA RBD DEQYJ SUT

AYNTMDBJQA ST DEQF. -DESJTDST UYVHQJ

328. FOB WEEU ZN L YZTS FOLF FLUBN MTLHB ZK

FOB SZKQ EY FOB JBLQBJ. FOLF'N AOD AB VE

FE SEXZBN LKQ NLD, "EO, FOB WEEU ZN

WBFFBJ." –MLGTE HEBTOE

329. FQ FT LSQQSX QU LS KMQSA NUX EKMQ RUV

MXS QKMG QU LS JUHSA NUX EKMQ RUV MXS

GUQ. – MGAXé PFAS, MVQVDG JSMHST

330. FQJF'O FQN JIJAPHK FQPHK JGYSF ISOPM:

FQNEN'O J OYHK LYE NXNEW NIYFPYH. MJH

WYS PIJKPHN J VYEUT VPFQ HY ISOPM? PF

VYSUT OSMD. -QJEEW OFWUNO

331. FTFDCYKOOL LUY PSOO IUQF CU

YDXFEZCKDX CWKC OUTF WFKOZ

FTFELCWSDM, KDX OUTF SZ KOO CWFEF SZ. -

MKEL HYRKT

332. FYNU VGP RSHN RPCWI GX FXWZN GX IXNSZN,

WZ'C XNSOOV VGPX DGQ ZG YSEN RWUM-

QOGFWUJ, WXXNCTGUCWQON, IGUMGRONCC

CNB FWZY FYSZNENX WMNS WZ WC VGP'XN

FXWZWUJ SQGPZ SZ ZYN ZWRN. -OSMV JSJS

333. G MH RF WFRDTY MOYMGN FO ETSFHGRD

WFUL, ETSMBUT LJT QFBYRTZ EMSP

MWCMZU YTKTMWU UFHTLJGRD RTC, MRN

LJML GU BWLGHMLTWZ DFFN OFY LJT

MYLGUL. — EGWWZ QFTW

334. GDF KUVTQ MZ GUU QWXIFVUBZ SUV

WXJGDMXI LBG GVBGD WXQ GUU ZAWTT SUV

WXJGDMXI LBG TUPF. -KMTTMWA ZTUWXF

RUSSMX

335. GFI JBYC GHTI DTHHIBDC SB GFSA

WPBUHTQG LJHYE...SA LFPG CJT AFPHI LSGF

AJRIJBI IYAI LFIB CJT'HI TBDJJY. -YIAGIH

WPBVA, PYRJAG XPRJTA

336. GFWQH QW PXYJSJY; GFWQH WBXFIR LYXM

NOR GNEFYJ MQEB CXF, PXIIXMQOL CXF

YQLBE XO FD FOEQI CXF RQJ. -DNFI WQGXO

337. GHBIJLHSZ LIISXZI XJLRBU HU CHWI

DFZZCHSZ DXBU RV SHLBR-ZCAJIBHSI:

ITMHCXBXLHSZ XSG GXSZIBRFU." — ULIOMIS

WHSZ

338. GHI NCL NY IJL FIIQPGHILK NY MNAL, MPWL

FQI, PK IN GQPCO JFQENCZ FCT NQTLQ NHI

NY UJFNK, IN PCIQNTHUL ELFCPCO FCT

FYYLUI BJLQL GLYNQL IJLQL BFK CNCL, IN

OPAL QJZIJEPU AFQPFIPNCK, JPOJK FCT

MNBK IN F MFCTKUFSL IJFI BFK

SQLAPNHKMZ YMFI. -ENMMZ JFKWLMM

339. GKDGEK CRX SK BDH P SCXK SYRPQ. P NKEE

NBKS P VYRN RNKG PTND PN. PN'R EPXK

RNKGGPTM PTND C OPIKO CTW VDPTPTM

NBK JEDH. KIKOF SDSKTN PT NBK OPIKO BCR

PNR RDTM. — SPQBCKE VCQXRDT

340. GKIKX LMXFGPID MAVITFAGFJ POF JKTI.

GKIKX MJ POF RFDNKBXL, POF FDFJ BXF POF

OBCCFXJ, POF JKTI MJ POF WMBAK HMPO

CBAD JPXMAZJ. POF BXPMJP MJ POF OBAL

POBP WIBDJ, PKTGOMAZ KAF RFD KX

BAKPOFX WTXWKJMYFID, PK GBTJF

YMNXBPMKAJ MA POF JKTI. -HBJJMID

RBALMAJRD

341. GL CJ ZW SLQJ ZM XJOJSB GL CJ ZW N

MGNGJ LD UJOEJUGANS NWJMGVJMZN – GL

XZMGNFJ NW LOTZWNOB BLAWP XNW DLO N

POJJF PLT LO NW LOTZWNOB BLAWP RLXNW

DLO N PLTTJMM. -V. S. XJWEFJW

342. GPO PH SDXJG DXS NPB SQSX CPYHC JP

SUEFDYH YH JSXTV PA WGSTYVJXN DHK

EGNVYWV VP YTEPXJDHJ D RYPFPCYWDF

EGSHPTSHPH DV AYXVJ FPQS? -DFRSXJ

SYHVJSYH

343. GQVLB LV E UEYHQEHJ KFEK WIJVY'K VRJEM

LY REDKLBQUED PIDWV. LK VRJEMV LY

JGIKLIYV, EYW LT LK'V LY KFJ OIYJV, LK'V

LY KFJ OIYJV. -MJLKF DLBFEDWV

344. GWXGEW UZS RW YXA H RUSW RBZHJ. H KWEE KYWR H LBZK ZKWG HVKX HK. HK'Z EHSW ZKWGGHVD HVKX U IHOWI UVN LXHVHVD KYW TEXA. WOWIQ RXRWVK HV KYW IHOWI YUZ HKZ ZXVD. -RHJYUWE LUJSZXV

345. GYL GTFON, LULDB KEB EN QLEZN, NG OLED E QXNNQL ZGYF, DLEK E FGGK RGLH, ZLL E JXYL RXVNTDL, EYK, XJ XN MLDL RGZZXWQL, NG ZRLEI E JLM DLEZGYEWQL MGDKZ. — CGOEYY MGQJFEYF UGY FGLNOL

346. GZIQ WU D SXZCWUQ, GZIQ WU D UZBIQEWX,

ZEOQ RWIQE EQIQX KZXRZJJQE, EQIQX GQJ

WJ PWUDSSQDX. -TZVE GQEEZE

347. H SUEKINU MGIM MGU LUIMKUX INU

FOMIWMX. JNPMPMQJUX PT UDPKOMHPWINQ

IBUWMX XUWM LQ BPS, UWSPRUS RHMG I

FQXMUNHPOX JPRUN MP ENUIMU I WUR

GOFIW XJUEHUX, I QPOWB NIEU PT

KIOBGHWB TNUUFUW. — MHFPMGQ KUINQ

348. H UXXL QHAADHUB DZ XVB CJDOJ HSSXCZ

RXA OJHVUB HVL UAXCKJ DV KJB

DVLDIDLGHSZ HVL DV KJB CHT KJBT

BMYABZZ KJBDA SXIB. -YBHAS Z. WGOF

349. HBGLGKMM BG TCILM UIKZSKM UCGPBLKGUK. HBGLGKMM BG SXBGHBGW UIKZSKM JICPQGLBSA. HBGLGKMM BG WBDBGW UIKZSKM YCDK. -YZC SOQ

350. HBIT RV R OBDTW XRU FB RUZDETWT. GS GVU'S VTUSGJTUSRH. GS QBTVU'S ERIT SB NT OWTSSZ, ZTS GS QBTVU'S QTUZ ORGU. -VERWBU VRHANTWF

351. HG XKR GWFGOMGRXG RSBTMRP YJB BTG FOGQGRB DSDGRB, IMEG MR RS SBTGO QGXSRN SV BMDG, KRN BS JRNGOQBKRN BTMQ MQ KQ XISQG KQ HG PGB BS GBGORKI IMVG. -F.N. LKDGQ, BTG XTMINOGR SV DGR

352. HGD TCYBOY B TGFFDESOH XSOZ FDWST, EGO

IDWO BO TGETYCOW PDO PH OBKJSEU

BPGDO SO XSOZ HGDC VCSYERW. -RBLSR

PHCEY

353. HMF PBTH FOWVHVIK NMEHMPT TFFP

ZIFOJFWHFL XIL WBPJGFO, HMF PBTH

AFXZHVDZG PFGBLVFT TVPJGF XIL

VIFQVHXAGF. -S.M. XZLFI

354. HMRY BRCC IL KOG GLACX HK TRKCLWUL: HK

VSNL VOYRU VKGL RWHLWYLCX, VKGL

ILSOHREOCCX, VKGL JLTKHLJCX HMSW LTLG

ILEKGL. -CLKWSGJ ILGWYHLRW

355. H'MX UYCUAZ BFNSKFB RXNRYX CNSYL JHWL

U YNB INEX RYXUZSEX HW BFXHE ENSBHWXZ

HJ BFXA QSEZB HWBN ZNWK UB

ZHKWHJHPUWB INIXWBZ. — DNFW

QUEENCIUW

356. HP'A AJUI Q UFTLYHUQPVR PIHWC PF LJP Q

TFMHV PFCVPIVX. PIV SFFN GFXYR HA AF

TJUI AHTLYVX. –QXPIJX AYQRV

357. HSNWV OSZUF NQ QD KMDQS GD HSNWV

MDCSF GOZG XDU GOS ZCSUZVS ISUQDW

GOSB ZUS ZMEDQG NWFNQGNWVJNQOZHMS.

-FZCNF ZJVQHJUVSU

358. HUL GT OML JU TYLXTRXUC EXLP IGTL

BXDXOB VMOUZ. VMOUZ XT OML UOMGBP,

VMOUZ AYO JU BML, JGL LPUZ OUUC ZMGW

PUYWLT LM HMDU LPUV. TM, TSWUYC ZMGW

HMDU UDUWZEPUWU ZMG BM. -VMLPUW

LUWUTY

359. HVPQ MLQB OVE GVS'Y SBBG YRB TVSBO.

MVUB MLQB OVE'UB SBUBP ZBBS REPY.

GXSWB MLQB SVZVGO'A HXYWRLSI. -

AXYWRBM KXLIB

360. HZTS, YS DSNHZPSX, FNJ KIQY HZWS N JLGV.

ZG UYS CSVZGGZGV UYSDS ZJ KOJUSDO, ZG

UYS SGX, UYSDS ZJ QLGTZDKNUZLG, CIU

ZU'J ZG UYS KZXXHS FYSDS NHH UYS

SKLUZLG DSJZXSJ UL KNWS UYS FYLHS

UYZGV FLDUYFYZHS. -GZQYLHNJ JRNDWJ

361. IC MIV EL ZCRVEZ VT FIC OVMCP FV TVPWERC

EL ZCRVEZ VT FIC OVMCP FV KVRC. FICPC EL

LVYC WVVZ EB FIC MVPLF VT DL QBZ LVYC

CREK EB FIC SCLF VT DL. MICB MC ZELNVRCP

FIEL, MC QPC KCLL OPVBC FV IQFC VDP

CBCYECL. -YQPFEB KDFICP GEBW HP.

362. ICJG FN XRG GALHSNFCS CT XPC SHXOUGN

FS NOZR THNRFCS XRHX GHZR FSZIOWG XRG

CXRGU, GHZR FN GSUFZRGW QM XRG CXRGU.

-TGIFA HWIGU

363. IFMU OUKTJSUT FJS TCKCJSU: CNU OFSU QU

IFMU, CNU PVEEUS QU KSU. CNUSU VT DF

TOKIIUS LKXRKEU VD KII CNU QFSIG CNKD

CNKC FB K OKD KII QSKLLUG JL VD NVOTUIB.

-QVIIVKO TIFKDU XFBBVD

364. IHUM NG CMUMF IHGB. NY CHB

FMWNXFHWOBMJ, NB ENII YIHE DOWV OCJ

GHYBMC OCJ XRFNYA BQM QMOFB. -

EOGQNCPBHC NFUNCP

365. IPNE QT IPPR EPC HJX TPWN. SPW IXH TP VFR

FH SPWCTXNE SPW EPCIXH HP JFHX SPWC

XLXVQXT. -OQNN CPIXCT

366. IWBDDFS JF, BQY U JBC QGD LFWUFNF CGH.

ASUDUAUVF JF, BQY U JBC QGD WURF CGH.

UMQGSF JF, BQY U JBC QGD IGSMUNF CGH.

FQAGHSBMF JF, BQY U XUWW QGD IGSMFD

CGH. WGNF JF BQY U JBC LF IGSAFY DG

WGNF CGH. -XUWWUBJ BSDEHS XBSY

367. J ITRA J'E CT CWYSJDGV LCZLG - J'E

CTWKRMJGZ. CTV TRL GMGDFPRVF ACTLZ

LKRZG KCJDF UJLLUG LKJTBZ. — LRDJ CERZ

368. J OIEJIZI BULB DTLCGIP BCDBU LTP

DTSNTPJBJNTLE ENZI MJEE ULZI BUI HJTLE

MNCP JT CILEJBA. BUJW JW MUA CJQUB,

BIGVNCLCJEA PIHILBIP, JW WBCNTQIC BULT

IZJE BCJDGVULTB. -GLCBJT EDBUIC YJTQ FC

369. JA XDOYP, NXMBX MR RE WQKK PE

ESDYWKENMCT, XOR EWPDC HDDC REKOBDG

OCG YDWYDRXDG HA JQRMB NXDC RMBF OCG

NDOYA. -JOYPMC KQPXDY

370. JANX DX PXNJUAMWX DCOZ MZ MR DX OPX

GXXVMAU, JANX DX PXNJUAMWX DX NOA

GXXV TXXQVF, VJEX TXXQVF, NOA GXXV LJF,

ZCXA DX DMVV TXBOAT ZCOZ OVV QOPZR JG

JSP VMEXR QPJTSNX ZCOZ IMAT JG LJF. -

OSTPX VJPTX

371. JBMSW SM EHBO HCL VAKVOSVLWV, EHBO

DTHBFTDM, EHBO CSMQHJ. SU EHB QHL'D

XSGV SD, SD CHL'D WHJV HBD HU EHBO

THOL. -WTYOXSV KYOIVO

372. JDI YBJJYI CEOIWIWHIOIK UGJP TQ FBEKEIPP

UEK YTLI UOI JDI HIPJ VUOJP TQ U VIOPTE'P

YBQI. -NBYYBUW NTOKPNTOJD

373. JGPNDCK GDUE YP TPPFK, NISXI GDUE YP

YISQFSQM UQE QPY YISQFSQM UQE YIDQ

LPCD JGPNDCK UQE LVKSX, LVKSX. YIDQ

LUQZ LPCD JGPNDCK UQE LUQZ LPCD TPPFK.

-LUSCU FUGLUQ

374. JKH'BD ZKQ QK UD BDPJ WIPDEHC AE JKH

SKG'Q VGKX XRDPD JKH IPD ZKAGZ,

UDWIHTD JKH FAZRQ GKQ ZDQ QRDPD. -JKZA

UDPPI

375. JMRKOKFKTO TR LTNC XTQLOZIKHB: EMTEIM

GUT NZO'F GLKFM, JTKOD KOFMLYKMGH

GKFU EMTEIM GUT NZO'F FUKOC, KO TLJML

FT ELMEZLM ZLFKNIMH RTL EMTEIM GUT

NZO'F LMZJ. — RLZOC AZEEZ, FUM LMZI

RLZOC AZEEZ PTTC

376. JNHU-HVBN LJ MVW JNHULJR; ZVG KIMMVW

WSGHZ HVBN IMVWRNS GMWLH ZVG FMVY

RVY WV HVBN ZVGSJNHU. -GMFMVYM

377. JP KTRJX JR Z CSZXL — OWLD BZYY JR OWL

XJOA, PMSN JR OWL UJSQLGDLRR, GMXN JR

OWL GMZQ, XSZRRJXZS JR Z OLKCSL. -ELGZ

DZYZGJZD

378. JQDV UQVNA'S KRNS NFS SEVLV JFIV C

NSQAV; FS ECN SQ MV HCUV, JFIV MLVCU,

LVHCUV CJJ SEV SFHV, HCUV AVT. -RLNRJC I.

JV ORFA

379. JS XSYP ICBSCOLJLSCQXXW UPZILUPM CS

BSCJUQBJM, AQUFQLCM, SU QFUPPKPCJM.

XSYP PELMJM LC JTP KSKPCJ-JS-KSKPCJ

HXIE SH XLHP. -KQULSC GSSOKQC

380. JT J FKM BA DJTU SH DJOU HOUG KPKJV, J

IHCDM FKOU BKMU K GCDU SH GUKM XHBU

LHUSGA KVM DJXSUV SH XHBU BCXJQ KS

DUKXS HVQU UOUGA IUUZ. -QFKGDUX

MKGIJV

381. K ALSE UJ URKOB ZOCJOS EJKOX ZOCURKOX

FSKHE FZL FSKHE. OJF K BOJF URZU KU KL

URS ISJIVS URZU TZVV JURSHL FSKHE URZU

ZHS FSKHE. -IZAV GTTZHUOSC

382. K PHD'Z ZQKDB UHI FSZ ZH FHHP VYKZKDF

IDCSOO UHI SLTHOS UHIYOSCA WDP UHIY

ASSCKDFO. PSST OHDFO PHD'Z NHES AYHE

ZQS OIYAWNS; ZQSU NHES AYHE ZQS PSST

PHVD. ZQS THSZYU WDP ZQS OHDFO ZQWZ

UHI WYS OITTHOSP ZH VYKZS, K JSCKSXS

WYS KD UHIY QSWYZ. -RIPU NHCCKDO

383. KI KD KM PHHT DZFKIBPH IGCI K WKMP IGH

AHMIFHMHDD RKIG RGKJG K JCM ISBFQ

FZOH UQ ESZIGHSD. IGH UZSH DZFKICSQ K

CU IGH UZSH CWWHJIKZM K GCOH WZS IGHU.

DZFKIBPH CMP DKFHMJH IHCJG UH IZ FZOH

UQ ESZIGHSD WZS RGCI IGHQ CSH, MZI WZS

RGCI IGHQ DCQ. -IGZUCD UHSIZ

384. **KLJP F YJGAVFM, F MJDJDTJM CLVC VXX**

CLMRBWL LFGCRMU CLJ KVU RN CMBCL VPY

XRZJ LVG VXKVUG KRP. CLJMJ LVZJ TJJP

CUMVPCG VPY DBMYJMJMG VPY NRM V CFDJ

CLJU GJJD FPZFPHFTXJ, TBC FP CLJ JPY,

CLJU VXKVUG NVXX – CLFPE RN FC, VXKVUG.

-DVLVCDV WVPYLF

385. **KR BCDVCHV ATKHNB ATOA ECWV OHJ**

MVOFV KB O FEKFTV ATOA DPBA TOWV GVVH

EVRA GVTKHJ KH ATV BKQAKVB, ATOA'B TKB

MUCGEVD. ECWV OHJ MVOFV OUV VAVUHOE.

-YCTH EVHHCH

386. KSUOE WGRFWUUWU DWWAOHQ CHV IBLSQBI,

TOIBLSI ACHQSCQW; OI TCU XWALT CHV

XWDLFW URWWEB, CHV OI OU CXLJW CHV

XWMLHV CAA TLFVU. -FLXWFI Q. OHQWFULAA

387. KTMBLW ZSIX ESSP DIXLCJ BLDS T OSMBC BQ

YBPC QCCBLW ZSIX SFCL DIXLCJ BLDS

ESIBYYSL GIECQ. –NSKL YC GTXXC

388. KU BJA'GH DOCKZX DKVQOCHV KQ DHOZV

BJA'GH JAQ QIHGH WJKZX VJDHQIKZX. –

ZHKM XOKDOZ, DOCH XJJW OGQ

389. KVOI MU ABL NOVULUA KSPL AV ABL KSPL DL

NSOO OMIL. EVT KLA RSH RYLSWU IYVP

KVVH UBVAU; EVT KLA KVVH RYLSWU IYVP

RSH UBVAU – RTA EVT BSJL AV FOSE ABL

RSOO DBLYL MA OMLU. -RVRRE QVZLU

390. KYNWRAXZXPP RP QFYYPRZW DY GYAX. RD

RP DFX KRNPD PORGG YK PXGK-WRARZW

GYAX. -BVFVDBV WVZIFR

391. KZZ WQQO RBLCMU KGQ UNCM. LR UQQIU

UNIQBNV RBQ FQGA HQCRGKZ QUUQCHQ ND

SU, UNCM; KU LD KZZ RBQ GQUR VQGQ TSR

VGKOOKMQU KCW BSZZU! -RBNIKU HKGZAZQ

392. L'R TLBYLUX YJ HAWIV BJJ ZYSZ RWBLH

ILKJB. OANJKJN. ZYSZ LZ'B BZNAUXJN ZYSU

VJSZY. BZNAUXJN ZYSU ZLRJ. SUV ZYSZ LZB

BZNJUXZY YAIVB DAW ZAXJZYJN TYJU

UAZYLUX JIBJ HSU. -MJUULOJN VAUUJIID

393. LEN, LENCFRMD, VF GNST VF VJLAEYL HJ QTR

RJQHCR NJHKRCFR, YRFRCKR LENC MEKR

VJY VDDRSQHEJ. -ANYYTV

394. LGPSW NASKFK. VQJ WGH OJCRF SF, VQNH

FQNEN GEN EGSHRJVK GHO VSIODIJVNEK,

FQN LCKSW JD FQN VSHO GHO FQN KSINHWN

JD FQN KFGEK? — HJEG EJRNEFK

395. LNR OZGCLR Z NRTAP OS WZAIL FUXR ILUAS –

Z ILTALRP FUUVZGM WUA SUC, GUL

VGUQZGM NUQ JFZGP LNTL QTI. FUXRAI

PUG'L WZGTFFS ORRL IUORQNRAR – LNRS'AR

ZG RTHN ULNRA TFF TFUGM. -ACOZ

396. LO KBC OUD QVQDPO L JDBFLGDI KUBO

QYCLZ ZBP IV OV XDVXFD, UVK LO ZBP QBWD

TVY UYJO BPI ADDF CV SVVI BFF BO VPZD. -

PLPB FBZVYJ

397. LSHEK EH PGY FIY EIKFBTFBYMX YIPBMIKY

EIPF PGY GEVGYB ZFBXC FO NIFZXYCVY

ZGEKG KFLTBYGYICH LMINEIC QSP ZGEKG

LMINEIC KMIIFP KFLTBYGYIC. -XSCZEV UMI

QYYPGFUYI

398. LSP JGBV HS, HGEV G TVVF CQVGHJ. GYT

GXXSR HJV DPNAM HS IXSR HJQSPWJ LSP.

QVBVX AY AH, GXXSR LSPQNVXI HS GRV.

RJVY LSP FXGL GXXSR HJV DPNAM HS CQVGE

LSPQ JVGQH RAHJ AHN CVGPHL. -EVXXL

RJAHV

399. LSVJ XGB LUJI YGOVISCJQ, UZZ ISV

BJCRVAYV EGJYHCAVY CJ SVZHCJQ XGB IG

UESCVRV CI. – HUBZG EGVZSG, ISV

UZESVOCYI

400. M RMC EU GSQDH ET FY EU ZFY TELUZ GVJY

VT M NVRMC. M NVRMC EU GSQDH ET UFY EU

ZFY GMUZ GVJY VT M RMC. -QFMLGYU

IEQDYCU

401. MD MHZU H VNNA UN VD H VNNA. MD'TT PHCD

HTT UPD LZUDEHSULCD VDTTK HZF

MPLKUTDK VIU NIE LZUDZU LK UN DZQHQD

XNIZQ RDNRTD LZ EDHFLZQ, ZNU UN KPNM

UPDG H GNCLD. –TDCHE VIEUNZ

402. MH CZH OYQP OBCO KHYKQH ROCF LT QYAH

JHNCIRH YD NBHELROZF, YZ JHNCIRH OBHF

ZHECLT LTOZLXIHP MLOB HCNB YOBHZ,

JHNCIRH YD ECTF GLTPTHRRHR, JHNCIRH YD

QING. JIO KCZO YD LO BCR XYO OY JH

DYZXLAHTHRR CTP XZCOHDIQTHRR. -HQQHT

XYYPECT

403. MJICGU, MFPUR, KJDIFR, WHRBV, CTIU PGI

CTI VGU JL CTI THWPK RMBGBC CGUBKO CJ

HKYIGRCPKY BCRIFL PKY WPQI RIKRI JL JHG

EJGFY. -F.W. IFFBJCC

404. MK SJQ QJE WTQMH. PTK MK SJNFE MKQ

QJERFQQ GMBF J PJKKGF VGJO. MK QJME

KUF TRMNFZQF UJE EXRF JGG MK HXTGE,

PTK DXT SFZF QKMGG JGMNF. — KFZZD

CZJKHUFKK, QXTG WTQMH

405. MKH EPTRJ YRHR OKJV FRIPLLPLI, MKH

XGTMHPVR QMQRLV YGJ HPIBV LMY, MKH

XGTMHPVR JMLIJ YRHR KLYHPVVRL. — HMF

JBRXXPRES, EMTR PJ G QPA VGUR

406. MN MW JFN Y QYKE FD QFZA, XPN Y QYKE FD

DHMAJGWIMR NIYN UYEAW PJIYRRV

UYHHMYOAW. -DHMAGHMKI JMANCWKIA

407. MNPYD ZNP BPTD QDDJBO RDTDF CFPZ PBQ;

MNDO KIO QUD PV PBQ ICD, SLM MNDO QUD

OPLRC. -YUF IFMNLF JURDFP

408. MPB OTA'J YDFYUD PTHD MPTJ JPDB MTAJ?

JPD JPGAWI MDQD TUU JPDQD JF OFAJDAJ

DHDQBEFZB; BDJ DHDQBEFZB PTI JPD

MQFAW JPGAW. KFQZ STZFL KFQZ, JPD WFFZ

IFUZGDQ

409. MPT IEOKW TUUTKMXOCU QH POYYXKTUU

OET: UQGTMPXKI MQ WQ, UQGTMPXKI MQ

CQNT, OKW UQGTMPXKI MQ PQYT HQE. -

OCCOK A. LPOCGTEU

410. MSLPSZMHV HEDV LEHHERK ZAV

CJMSNMCHV: 'M HEDV UVNPGKV M PQ

HEDVF.' QPZGJV HEDV LEHHERK ZAV

CJMSNMCHV: 'M PQ HEDVF UVNPGKV M

HEDV.' MQQPZGJV HEDV KPBK: 'M HEDV BEG

UVNPGKV M SVVF BEG.' QPZGJV HEDV KPBK:

'M SVVF BEG UVNPGKV M HEDV BEG.' -VJMNA

LJEQQ

411. MVD HPFD PE PGO KDNQVLPO NK BHH NMU

EGHHKDUU UNJCHZ JDBKU LDNKQ BLHD MP

UBZ, 'AVBM BOD ZPG QPNKQ MVOPGQV?' -

UNJPKD ADNH

412. MZIPW GNIZT: H FHFI'R SINB WNQ YNQJF XJW

K LJKIZ! HIFHKIK GNIZT: XJW -- WZT, JKIF --

IN. — PNC EKYAPZANP, HIFHKIK GNIZT KIF

RMZ JKTR YPQTKFZ

413. NC DFF UCCE ZKVCUEH NVLQ NQRP NC IDU

HOCDG RZ RBK ECCOCHL IRUICKUH, DUE NQR

ER URL ZCDK LR HOCDG LQC LKBLQ VU FRAC

LR BH. -PDKTDKCL TBCULQCK

414. NFJ NHGJP AQC DHWJT NFZQCYF, NFJ

SJQSDJ AQC PFEZJT NFQPJ NHGJP OHNF –

LQNFHLY VZHLYP HN EDD NQ DHRJ DHMJ EL

QDT GHB NESJ. HN TQJP E VJNNJZ IQV QR

PNQZHLY CS GJGQZHJP NFEL EUNCED VZEHL

NHPPCJ UEL TQ. -ZQV PFJRRHJDT

415. NJX WGROP XLPJTLNXQ NJX TOC. ON BTR

VODX NJX RHGNJ BOLQ, VODX T BTCW

LOMJN, VODX RBXVVOLM RTOVR SXLXTNJ

NJX RNTCR, PHWYVXNXVZ TLQ GNNXCVZ

GLCXTV... -XCOPJ WTCOT CXWTCKGX

416. NJY YKJ NEGJP QJ RFDHPLUJTON, UPLBA,

LQDJSY-XFSRJR. DEXJESJ DEQJP MFNN

MEPPA LQEOY JGJSYD HEFSH QLRNA. NJY

YKJ NEGJP QJ. -POXF

417. NL SVVH BVKNFKM XV XQL XZWL NQLJ XQL

CVNLK VB SVRL NZSS KLCSFDL XQL SVRL VB

CVNLK. XQLJ NZSS VYK NVKSM HJVN XQL

PSLEEZJIE VB CLFDL. -NZSSZFW L.

ISFMEXVJL

418. NPQ IDP MBDA INKQRA, FON DZQ ZQCVTZQR

HNZ KQBNRZDKD, YVF D FZDXQRA RQKDPRE

FWZQQ. -QBYQZF WVYYDZR

419. NQ N LDFRHG UWUZ GNU, JFG QFZCNG, HUP

PDNL CU BE UINPTID: 'PDU FOHE IZFFQ DU

OUUGUG QFZ PDU USNLPUOVU FQ JFG KTL

BRLNV'. -MRZP WFOOUJRP

420. NRC L JPO BDC LB CIH NPBS, NHFPROH L

ORWWHQ WQDE CIH ULBS DW CDBH-

SHPWBHOO CIPC LO YHBHQPVVG

POODFLPCHS JLCI PFCRPV SHPWBHOO. —

XDIB YQHHB, APAHQ CDJBO

421. NRJP JQKIYTWBPW ATXP. AR NRJPEW, Q

XRXPKA UQK MP PAPEKTAF, PAPEKTAF UQK

MP ABP ATUC RG Q UNRUC. -XQEF OQEETWB

422. NS YKCQMS BD XD YKCQFHLDD XD MRL DLX.

NS HKZL XD FLLJ; MRL NKOL B IBZL MK

MRLL. MRL NKOL B RXZL, GKO YKMR XOL

BQGBQBML. -PBHHBXN DRXWLDJLXOL

423. NTVEB LTTAPW PDUTL NW HDITDET BVUTH

WDC HGKTEBGQ, MQVPT PDUVEB HDITDET

LTTAPW BVUTH WDC RDCKOBT. -POD GSC

424. NWGRJ GYFWSI GOTRQL CRTL CTFN OYL

YLVTO FC NVX, VXI ETRXK OLVTG CTFN OYL

LALG FC BFNVX. -SWIBRK UVX ELLOYFULX

425. NXFDWZ NJLUIW YJC J BWSZ PQQG PQIMWS,

KRU YW YWSWL'U JIIQYWG UQ OIJZ PQIM

GRSXLP UVW CWJCQL; QLIZ JU COSXLP

USJXLXLP. -ZQPX KWSSJ

426. NXKG GDYE KG TDL NXV EJB HXD MVVZG

BVWWKYE TLDR NXV ACWSDYB, CYQ KN'G

SCWWVQ, 'HV XCNV BDJ, ZWVCGV QKV. -

ALBCY WVV D'RCWWVB, GSDNN ZKWELKR

427. O CNUOWTD OUN – GMCBX – NID GFCN

VFDNBX OWJ VUDXBCD FR OEE NID OUNC,

POTMD OC O JUDOG OWJ VUDXBCD OC

OETDLUO. -TMA JD GOMVOCCOWN

428. O EWWN RDTOI. OV'T MOZW RB QWLJVXWLV,

TP VP TUWLZ. OV ZWWUT RW APOEA EP

RLVVWJ HQLV'T APOEA PE – XLN ALRWT,

UJWTT, HQLVWFWJ! -MWXJPE GLRWT

429. OCHJ MCJV RCN YCRVEVN CT BFAERB FN

JFYU CNUJW, KGN ER OCCLERB NCBJNUJW

ER NUJ VFQJ MEWJYNECR. -FRNCERJ MJ

VFERN-JZGIJWP

430. OED KGBNFZ LP QDQKDGZ LP OED SGDZZ

IDSBGOQDFOZ LP QLONLF-SNJORGD ZORINLZ

GDZDQKYD ZLRS BO B JEDBS GDZOBRGBFO.

NO NZ XNZDG FLO OL ZONG OEDQ." — S.T.

XLIDELRZD

431. OGMQ K GMDJ YTLKR, K IMDJ QP BDQZMJ. K DY KQNTSQMJDESM. K LMM QP IPM. K DY JMSDWMB WP WGM MDJSKMLW WKYML, DQB WP WGM SDWMLW. -GMQJV BDNKB WGPJMDT

432. OIRMR FMR QJO LJMR OIFQ SCNR LKYCXFZ QJORY, WRO OIR XJLHCQFOCJQY JS OIRYR SCNR TCNR MCYR OJ LJMR LRZJPCRY OIFQ XFQ RNRM HR IRFMP. -YKQ OUK

433. OL DXYYUT IPL IU XTU, OL DXYYUT IPXY LMT

NWTNMDJYXONUJ, LMT SUUGWOVJ XOB

UDLYWLOJ XTU MOWZUTJXG. XOB DMJWN

PXJ XGIXAJ QUUO X VTUXY IXA YL DXFU

CULCGU XIXTU LS YPXY NLOOUNYWLO. -HLJP

VTLQXO

434. OS LBXZB GL EHKKC BZDKOYZ ALN VDX D

ILIHKDB IKDC JDS VZ, OG OT SZJZTTDBC GL

TZZ OG GNOJZ. -WZLBWZ VZBSDBX TADN

435. OSBP MF BMDH G BSWH GPPGMT. MP RSA

ISU'K KGDH MK FHTMSAFBR, MK'F US PAU;

MP RSA IS KGDH MK FHTMSAFBR, MK QTHGDF

RSAT LHGTK. -GTKLAT IGBHR

436. P BRQ GYOE BPDS UTQPA PEQPKM UM. UTQPA

BRQ YEM YJ UF CRODQ. XPWM UF OPGQ, UF

WPKEMFQ, UF XPIMO, UF SMROD. XPWM UF

GXYYK. PD BRQ R JYOAM RXOMRKF BPDSPE

UM BSME P ROOPIMK YE DSM QAMEM. PD BRQ

R EMAMQQPDF JYO UM – XPWM JYYK YO

BRDMO. -ORF ASROXMQ

437. P IKLKU OSWDK DRMKSB ZNKI P'D IFV

NPVVPIQ. P GAMV OSWDK VNK OWV WIY PB

PV HKKJM AJ, P ENWIQK OWVM. WBVKU WSS,

PB P HIFZ PV PMI'V DR BWASV VNWV P'D IFV

NPVVPIQ, NFZ EWI P QKV DWY WV DRMKSB? -

RFQP OKUUW

438. PF SMMT PGO LVGY VYN SAIYFN GS GYSM OMCFSPGYD HFVASGQAK. GYSM OMCFSPGYD SPVS LFMLKF WMYYFWS SM. VYN SPVS'O UPVS DMMN CAOGW NMFO. GS OLFVTO SM RMA. GS WPVYDFO RMA. -PVYYVP PVIIGYDSMY

439. PF XNKI NC PF MI VACNRZX, CPZWPNDH QNPJ PJI MXFFO OZDRNDH ND SFAW KINDC. IKIWSPJNDH XNKNDH JZC Z WJSPJV. OF SFA LIIX SFAW VACNR? -VNRJZIX UZRGCFD

440. PFA, LFSSFO, EZVSL, JVHZBEVEUFB,

JVMKQEZS – EF VJJ EQZLZ HMLUR KUTZL

TFURZ, IME UB LMRQ V OVA EQVE OZ VSZ

ESVBLDFSEZC WSFH EQZ OFSJC FW MBSZLE

EF V OFSJC FW DZVRZ... -VJIZSE

LRQOZUEYZS

441. PI AFXRV'I YMIIXL PW INX QEU PR CXLWXHI FL

INX QPLD PR CXLWXHI, MR DFVQ MR INXU

MLX CXLWXHI WFL XMHN FINXL. -RXMV (QFFA

TPDD NEVIPVQ)

442. PJAC FML CACH ICCW DW BMAC? PMHHDIBC

DTW'O DO? DO EJQCT FML TM ALBWCHJIBC.

DO MXCWT FMLH GPCTO JWR DO MXCWT LX

FMLH PCJHO JWR DO ECJWT OPJO TMECMWC

GJW UCO DWTDRC FML JWR ECTT FML LX. -

WCDB UJDEJW

443. PKLUQ EDF LUSMDQM QNPHUDM LOWNDRSA

HMQEKLM PKLUQ UL FNDM JUOV LUSMDQM,

EDF LUSMDQM UL ZKSS NZ PKLUQ. -PEWQMS

PEWQMEK

444. PMHSJ... BSAA CWAF USHHKAIW EKMV

FWVFAWGSDSWH LZU FMVSXE EKMV

JCLVLJDWV LZU HWZHSRSASDSWH, LZU SZ

DSPW KX JLVW LZU HKVVKB, BSAA YWWF L

XKMZDLSZ KX QKE LASIW SZ EKM. -

USWDVSJC RKZCKWXXWV

445. PMWR PYKR TSU PYKR QYPP PMWR CMD

JTNB. PMWR ZRMZPR TSU FIRC QYPP PMWR

CMD JTNB. -TGFIDG GDJYSHFRYS

446. PO JUPERIDH UDQI OPHD XMCPJ OIYX VUD RQN YO VUDPI GPIVU QHR EDQIH VY LEQN PV, VUDN RDKDEYL CDHCPVPKPVN, RPCJPLEPHD, QHR DHRMIQHJD. VUDN BDV Q GDQMVPOME UDQIV. -CUPHPJUP CMWMFP

447. PR PIBLDM QU BD BJOI BLI HBPDUB BEDHSZI BD CQTM BLI EQKLB BLQTK BD UJR, JTM BLIT BD UJR QB GQBL BLI HBPDUB ZIWQBR. - KIDEKI SIETJEM ULJG

448. PUF BLFWPFZP CFBLFF GM JSSFL

PLWSXIJEJPT DGQFZ MLGQ PUF

CFAFEGYQFSP GM EGAF WSC DGQYWZZJGS.

PUF QGLF NF DWLF MGL PUF UWYYJSFZZ GM

GPUFLZ, PUF BLFWPFL JZ GIL GNS ZFSZF GM

NFEE-KFJSB. -CWEWJ EWQW

449. Q EXGOKM XY ZOXGRWM LE XGO GJOGWC

HLJNE. UM KQJ KXGJZMO ZDQZ RC

NMPMWXILJF Q UQOH DMQOZ. UM JMMN ZX

MYYMKZ QJ LJJMO ZOQJEYXOHQZLXJ, ZX

GJNMOEZQJN ZDQZ WXPM QJN QYYMKZLXJ

QOM Q OMQW EXGOKM XY TXC. -NQWQL

WQHQ

450. QBDW DW TFYL: QF GTA QFKMNS M WLJNLQ

WHA, QF JMOWL M BORSNLS YLDTW QF GMTT

LMJB XFXLRQ. GDNWQ QF TLQ IF FG TDGL.

GDRMTTA, QF QMHL M WQLC KDQBFOQ GLLQ.

-NOXD

451. QCH OVTIQ IQHF – HIFHXVWAAZ OMT ZMBSJ

FHMFAH NVQC HSHTJZ WSG GTVUH WSG

QWAHSQ, RBQ SMQ YMSHZ – QCH OVTIQ IQHF

QM XMSQTMAAVSJ ZMBT NMTAG VI QM

XMSQTMA ZMBT XBAQBTH. QM NTVQH QCH

RMMEI. YWEH QCH YBIVX. ICMMQ QCH OVAYI.

FWVSQ QCH WTQ. -XCBXE FWAWCSVBE

452. QCSY DNAX UJFAVP, ECI UJYIYFA QFYP UJY

UILY PUIYAVUJ, NAM ZJCPCYSYI QCSYP

DLWJ GYIECIDP DLWJ, NAM WNA

NWWCDGQFPJ DLWJ, NAM ZJNU FP MCAY FA

QCSY FP MCAY ZYQQ. -SFAWYAU SNA VCVJ

453. QFGON HVJXVNHG KJH HUFNXKOWV WB WFZ

NJOCUZHV PT JHCEOVY KJHQ KW QXIH

NWVVHNKOWVG XVU PZWXUHVOVY KJH

UHEKJ SOKJ SJONJ KJHT KJOVI XVU BHHC. -

TW-TW QX

454. QGQMACUSA TYI VTYV FUEKV EK VTQEM

NEDQ HTQMQ AUW TEV Y OMUIIMUYSI YKS

AUW'GQ TYS Y CWKOT UD CYS SYAI YKS

VTQMQ'I SEDDQMQKV HYAI AUW OYK SQYN

HEVT EV YKS VTQ HYA E SQYNV HEVT EV HYI

E XWIV VWMKQS OULFNQVQNA VU LWIEO. —

VYANUM IHEDV

455. QGT KJOYQ YLFCQSF SK VSZT JP N LSMPH

FNP JY QJFJIJQL; JP N HJOV WSVIPTYY. -

ZJUQSO GMHS

456. QHE UYZYN JHOY MQ JHZTUR. QHE XJVXQO

JHOY MQ FHJCTUR MXWA. -MXNMXNX CY

XURYJTO

457. QR MPP GRRW ZLYRGWT QYOD QDFB QR HMG TURMI FZ FVL WRRURTO HFGHRLGT, MGW QDF WF GFO ZRML OF TURMI ODR OLVOD YG PFNR OF VT. -BMLKMLRO KVRGODRL

458. QS EPB IQAZ JP XZ W MBCVFZV, Q GWCJ JP IQAZ JP XZ W MBCVFZV OQCBL PCZ VWE LP Q CZAZF MWAZ JP IQAZ GQJMPBJ EPB. -W. W. OQICZ

459. QV CHYRI'V GBVVYE KPH AHW BEY HE KPBV AHW THHU TQUY, RH THIX BR RHGYFHCA THSYR AHW. -EHBTC CBPT, VPY KQVLPYR

460. QVC QRGQ KTBVNKL RB RHH, SDB QNYJHG QBRWCQ DJARWP NKBT BVC PRWE QEG RKP ARBOVCQ, ANBV QRP CGCQ, BVC QHTA PRKOC TX BVC NKXNKNBC QBRWQ. -KCNH LRNYRK, QBRWPDQB

461. QVFG, OUFLXP XV PGVPNUBOD, IXVRH XV SVMXWUNLGH: RGLPOZ UXW HLXI LZ WGGB, XV EUZZGN, LZ RLQQ NLHG UXW CLXW ZOG HMNCUKG. -ZNMEUX KUBVZG

462. QVY'IT OVAAS USRWT KFMT ALTHT'C RVEVUQ

PSAWLFRO, KVIT KFMT QVY'KK RTITH ET

LYHA, CFRO KFMT ALTHT'C RVEVUQ

KFCATRFRO, SRU KFIT KFMT FA'C LTSITR VR

TSHAL. -PFKKFSX P. BYHMTQ

463. QWZ RDZV LDG JHDGZFG ADE CHDI MDTZ,

NEG MDTZ GD VDIZ ZKGZLG JHDGZFGV ADE

CHDI QWZ. -XZQLLZ IDHZQE

464. **QX SCW RNZNBCL FK NFG XCG UCWKRU IEFI**

FGN JWUQYFB QI QU BQON RNZNBCLQKT FK

NTC. SCW VNTQK IC GNXWUN UCWKRU IEFI

FGN KCI JWUQYFB FKR IEFI MFS YWI

SCWGUNBX CXX XGCJ F TCCR RNFB CX

NPLNGQNKYN. — DCEK YFTN

465. **R LMEBZK BU LWRBZ MEK KRWZJB AUTRZN**

MEK EUB CZ QUWJZK BU MKMSB BOZA QWUA

M CZNBNZVVRED CUUH. –QWMEJRN QUWK

JUSSUVM

466. R PYQV RL LKEO, GPMLOJOK XOBMQQ; R

BOOQ RL, GPOA R UYKKYG HYUL; 'LRU

XOLLOK LY PMJO QYJOV MAV QYUL LPMA

AOJOK LY PMJO QYJOV ML MQQ. -MQBKOV

LOAAZUYA

467. R TDBU ODY PDL DPTO EDH ZFXL ODY XHU,

GYL EDH ZFXL R XS ZFUP R XS ZRLF ODY. R

TDBU ODY PDL DPTO EDH ZFXL ODY FXBU

SXNU DE ODYHIUTE, GYL EDH ZFXL ODY XHU

SXVRPW DE SU. R TDBU ODY EDH LFU QXHL

DE SU LFXL ODY GHRPW DYL. -UTRJXGULF

GXHHULL GHDZPRPW

468. **R XSJN VQWRS ON YRQFBMC JMB HSVB JQU**

CWRYY YMLO WIB KLSU, JQU WIBQ R GBBX

LQ XSJNRQF. VQWRS R'O SLCW RQ WIB

OVCRK. VQWRS R JO WIB OVCRK – QLWBC

JQU KILMUC, WIB OBSLUN JQU IJMOLQN. -

PBQQRYBM ULQQBSSN

469. **RAALW UPG BADCIW UJI SCLI UMMSIW UPG**

AJUPYIW. OQIX RAOQ UJI KJVCO, RVO OUWOI

TABMSIOISX GCKKIJIPO. –WOIMQIP LCPY

470. RARYJEO XYJNYOL HP E RJEXL MFLOL RHNZ

HP XEJJLU XACREPPHAK, GJENNLOZ HP

XEJJLU JASL, ROAREDEKUE HP XEJJLU

IKAMJLUDL, NLKPHAK HP XEJJLU RLEXL,

DAPPHR HP XEJJLU KLMP, EKU EYNA-NYKL

HP XEJJLU PHKDHKD. — XOHPP TECH,

IHJJAPARFZ

471. RDDORW ZORN ZLOS FYQ RWO GJWYSX, RST

GJWYSX ZLOS FYQ RWO ZORN. – GQS JAQ,

JLO RWJ YV ZRW

472. RGQ LCTQ DIYQT RCADTFK RGQ SDKR XCP

VDTTX OI XCPT GQDTR, RGQ WQKK VDSDZWQ

XCP DTQ CN WCHOIY OI RGQ STQKQIR. -

ZDTZDTD FQ DIYQWOK

473. RGWVW OJ I KILQWJJ OQ YBEOQD SBT, I YINX

BM VWIJBQ RGIR KIXWJ OR MWWY JB

MYICYWJJ. -YWB NGVOJRBZGWV

474. RJZC AJCU KJP LCQXK MKA CKA PWC GMS GC

UCCH PJ PWXKE XP AJCU. RJZC XU M

LMPPRC, RJZC XU M GMN; RJZC XU M

QNJGXKQ TI. -VMHCU LMRAGXK

475. **RLIEQO WHQ ALK OUHEFKO – RLIEQO WHQ TEGRO; KJQP'HQ ALK NLLMO, KJQP'HQ ALK KJQ KJQWKHQ. –AEULGWO HLQC**

476. **RNED QV YNCD ZGMA M ANSA – QZ QV M EDCP; QZ QV YNCD ZGMA M UDDRQAT – QZ QV BMCQAT, VGMCQAT, GDROQAT, VMBCQUQBQAT. -JQRRQMY MCZGSC JMCW**

477. RQDS HSDSJ PGSF N HNBVJNR PSNBA. GB

PGSF ISENVFS US PQH'B YHQU AQU BQ

JSCRSHGFA GBF FQVJES. GB PGSF QM

IRGHPHSFF NHP SJJQJF NHP ISBJNTNRF. GB

PGSF QM GRRHSFF NHP UQVHPF; GB PGSF QM

USNJGHSFF, QM UGBASJGHKF, QM

BNJHGFAGHKF. -NHNGF HGH

478. RQZFS HXFCIZ KWQ. FL MONIZ KWQ QA, FL

EILZ KWQ AQRAFGE. OGH, OL LUI IGH WD LUI

HOK, LUI SWXXISL LQGI MFBB SUFBB KWQ

HWMG. -HFRIJOE HOXXIBB

479. RXO EHWZ VS EHKVTN XIJAK KH GIFX? RZ

EHWZ AH MTHR AXQA RZ QJZ THA QEHTZ. -F.

K. EZRVK

480. RY R ZQDQ LWJ O TICMRNRMJ, R ZWFVG

TDWEOEVC EQ O XFMRNROL. R WYJQL JIRLS

RL XFMRN. R VRKQ XC GOCGDQOXM RL

XFMRN. R MQQ XC VRYQ RL JQDXM WY

XFMRN. -OVEQDJ QRLMJQRL

481. RZGCN JHZNLYCDX DUJXG HDDPG YWLY

WJEU NWCEHPJX ULGG APDR GNWDDE CXYD

YWJ MDPEH LPDZXH YWJR – L MDPEH DA

MDPS, NZEYZPJ, CXYJEEJNYZLE LNYCQCYO,

LXH WZRLX CXQDEQJRJXY. -FJPLEH P. ADPH

482. S ZMSDB ZMG PSLLGYZ VSYGRYG ZMG AKJEV

YWUUGJY UJKF SD ZMSY VRX RDV RLG SY

ZMG VSYGRYG KU NGKNEG UGGESDL

WDEKCGV. -NJSDHGYY VSRDR

483. S ZSLO IYIVGXPWG OUW DOI WVSYI OI (QPI

WSAUJJSP) OUW. OI CIYIV WSW UCGDOSCJ

ZVPCJ PC DOI RSIHW. S'W CIYIV LIIC OSA

WSYI RPV U XUHH, IYIVGDOSCJ ZUL U NOILD-

OSJO NUDNO, UCW OI CIYIV ZUHEIW PRR DOI

RSIHW. -GPJS XIVVU

484. S'B PQM CUVSPF S'B FQPPU JDUPFI MDI

NQOTX, YGM S FGUOUPMII MDUM S NSTT

CWUOR MDI YOUSP MDUM NSTT JDUPFI MDI

NQOTX. -MGWUJ CDURGO

485. S'TV JYGV RY RNV JYWJKAISYW RNDR

LVYLKV PNY PVDO NVDBLNYWVI PNSKV

RNVZ PDKH DOV GAJN NDLLSVO, GYOV

JYWMSBVWR, DWB GYOV UVDARSMAK

SWBSTSBADKI RNDW IYGVYWV GDHSWC RNV

IYKSRDOZ BOABCV RY PYOH PSRNYAR

DJHWYPKVBCSWC RNVSO YPW SWRVOVIRI

DWB LYPVO. — QDIYW GODX

486. S'Z HJKHBT VIXTUIHUWQ KPWG TMZWRMQB

ZHAWT H ZMCSW MXU MV H RMMA HGQ UPWB

JWHCW UPW RMMA RWPSGQ, MI UPW PWHIU

MV SU. –TWHG EWGG

487. SBY GFRQP HB IOFRL CS IOFRLMPJ, HB IHYVS

CS IHYVSMPJ, HB QYP CS QYPPMPJ, HB ABQL

CS ABQLMPJ; RPV NYIH IB, SBY GFRQP HB

GBTF CS GBTMPJ. RGG HUBIF AUB HUMPL HB

GFRQP MP RPS BHUFQ ARS VFXFMTF

HUFZIFGTFI. -IRMPH KQRPXMI VF IRGFI

488. SCNK SN PNNX XHEN OKU DGKUKNRR

JHSOBUR HJCNBR, GJ KHJ HKXZ YODNR

HJCNBR PNNX XHENU OKU MOBNU PHB, QLJ

GJ CNXFR LR OXRH JH UNENXHF GKKNB

COFFGKNRR OKU FNOMN. -UOXOG XOYO

489. SDXDV TFJD KCTDCSD F IVMCVMRH UYDS FZZ

HCA FVD RC RYDT MK FS CIRMCS. -TFHF

FSNDZCA

490. SELC Y UX ... WJXFVLRLVZ XZHLVD,

LCRYMLVZ UVJCL... JM GQMYCB REL CYBER

SELC Y WUCCJR HVLLF, YR YH JC HQWE

JWWUHYJCH REUR XZ YGLUH DVJS TLHR

UCG XJHR UTQCGUCRVZ. SELCWL UCG EJS

RELHL YGLUH WJXL Y PCJS CJR CJM WUC Y

DJMWL RELX. — SJVDBUCB UXUGLQH

XJAUMR

491. SFWHB XEW E RNOQK NJ JNKSHCD UXQ

BXEKEBUQK, ECL WXNFML UXQKQJNKQ IQ

HCUKNLFBQL HCUN UXQ QLFBEUHNC NJ UXQ

PNFCD. -EKHWUNUMQ

492. SI S HC LBN ABVNR NRK ABBSLO, S HC

FYVKUG LBN ABVNR NRK ASLLSLO. -RKLVG

AHJFABVNR UBLOIKUUBA

493. SKSG KR YI XGJEEA DWJSPGI KZGX VUTG. BG

KSEA NGDKTG TKXG RYEEA BWJV BG JXG. –

JSSG XUDG, VWG ZJTQUXG EGIVJV

494. SL EQ CLAU YUMQDX KRN RHH M QZQU

KRDSQX; SL EQ CLAU HLZQU KRN RHH M

QZQU XUQRTQX. -ZRHQUMQ HLTERUXL

495. SM NZ ELSMSEM, HPP NBM HTB SWPHMUW.

HMU FVHR'W NETB, MEF'W RVB RSNB RE JB

EMB. RVSW SW HM SWPHMU HKB. -FSPP,

HJEYR H JEZ

496. SPA SCFA LATFSM ZU WFYHG HY SPTS HS GZVVAGSY KAZKEA. HS GTCCHAY T WAYYTDA, TVI BA, SPA WFYHGHTVY, TCA SPA WAYYAVDACY. -CZM TMACY

497. SPEWB EHLKPFL IPNW HG BWXZIWGG JOY JDFGHNW, JOY IPNW EHLKPFL SPEWB HG GWOLHRWOLJI JOY JOWRHX. -RJBLHO IFLKWB ZHOM CB.

498. SQ YSQL SPD ZGQJ QZ VBYRH JQBGX UD GROD SPD YSQLLREK QZ SRVD RSYDGZ, REHWDXRUGD CEX REHQEHDRFCUGD. — CCWQE HQLGCEX

499. SRVJFUELSJR SM RJL ZRJPXHQCH.

ZRJPXHQCH SM RJL PSMQJU. PSMQJU SM

RJL LFTLA. LFTLA SM RJL NHETLB. NHETLB

SM RJL XJOH. XJOH SM RJL UTMSD. UTMSD

SM LAH NHML. -VFERZ YEKKE

500. ST YDDE SGW BIGV IVN YZMVTN GY GVYD

WDCTYSGVP OTIZYGRZK. GVYD WDCTYSGVP

YSIY BTDBKT LDVVTLY YD. IVN YSIY'W FSIY

PDDN CZWGL NDTW. GY WBTIEW YD QDZ. GY

LSIVPTW QDZ. — SIVVIS SIMMGVPYDV,

WIXGVP HZVT

501. SW XRAV RJ SW DV NEJRITX, JSTMSRHO PRSF

SFV DXWWQ QTHIRHO RH GWEM AVRHJ.

VAVMGSFRHO XRARHO FTJ T MFGSFN. QW

GWE CVVX GWEM NEJRI? — NRIFTVX BTILJWH

502. SYMP BIEP NG XISC BIENQU HQW BPSSNQU

IQPGPBR XP BIEPW. NS NG CHYWPY SI BPS

IMYGPBEPG XP BIEPW SCHQ NS NG SI BIEP. -

JIJP RYHQDNG

503. SYN NFJXNJS EFA SU FGUXQ EDUVP VUSNJ

XJ SU VNGND UMNV AUWD IUWSY FVQ JXVP.

EYFS F IXJSFRN SYFS EUWBQ CN. -MNSN

JNNPND

504. T NXR EKXE VQB ROPO UOPSOHE, XDW NQ T

FQZOW VQB. EKOD T NXR EKXE VQB ROPO

DQE UOPSOHE XDW T FQZOW VQB OZOD

LQPO. -XDMOFTEX FTL

505. T XFNRZF CM IFKTFJF CPGC PFLQXTE PGQ

CPF KGZC VMZZFZZFQ PGLQ, CPGC HMVKTL

PGQ CPF KGZC QXRLWFL CPXMGC, CPGC

BMXXTZML PGQ CPF KGZC FLKTDPCFLFQ

BTLQ. — VGCCT ZBTCP

506. T'Q HGP MGTHM PG EVZ QZ FTWY CH

JHIZIDGNJWTC. DJP PRJQ ACDF PG YIRGGD

DTFJ T WTW. -ZGMT EJOOC

507. TDYK IDNKPGNKI ABJPI PD ED LI B HCKBP

QBYDC: MDTE LI LWIGEK EDAJ BJE IMBFK

BTT PMK JDJIKJIK DLP. -MBQGR DQ WKCIGB

508. THAJP – OBNO'A DVVU TF VZHPNOJQU.

OBVLV'A UQO N ZNF OBNO EQVA DF OBNO J

ONYV JO SQL ELNUOVZ. -DJCCJV IQV

NLTAOLQUE

509. TI VWLE QHH NQMI EDI MDJRMI PIETIIZ TDQE

RL URFDE QZG TDQE RL IQLA. – C.B. UJTHRZF,

DQUUA OJEEIU QZG EDI FJPHIE JN NRUI

510. TJ THOPV DPKK WA AF MASRXRS. TIJCR PU'O I MAAK OIJ UBIU, CHU DBRF TR YFAD MIVUO TR VIF OIJ MIVUO. TJ THOPV DPKK WA AF MASRXRS. -CAC TISKRJ

511. TM OMF SMXI ZI UIRVFPI Q'Z UIVFHQEFS, MD VZ Q UIVFHQEFS UIRVFPI OMF SMXI ZI? - MPRVD CVZZIDPHIQG

512. TZ IXH FOVPT ADFA L'T KQXFALIE, HDLKD LC JLILCDXG YQXAAZ TPKD, HFC HQLAAXI HLAD ADLC IXH LICALIKAPFO XIXQEZ ADFA L'UX GXUXOBYXG EXAALIE AB WIBH TZ JFIC. ADXZ YQBAXKA TX, CB IBH LA'C TZ GXCALIZ AB YQBAXKA ADXT. — OFGZ EFEF

513. U JHSBRBGTD UZUMHWBWR ZQBFQ XGHD

WGP UZUMHW PQH DSHHAHJ PG SGIH QUD

JGTDHX QBE BW IUBW. -NHDDUEOW ZHDP

514. U ROUS VINAOZ WKPF SNA VNQFEIKCW EN

EIKCJ UHNAE. GIFC K VFF U ROUS UCZ

ACZFTVEUCZ KE EIF BKTVE EKQF, EIFC K

JCNG KE XUC'E HF QAXI WNNZ. -E. V. FOKNE

515. UDH KOLZC QOL QCNC ZCCD HUDESDV QCNC

KOLBVOK KL PC SDZUDC PA KOLZC QOL

ELBMH DLK OCUN KOC IBZSE. -GNSCHNSEO

DSCKRZEOC

516. UE YH GEKHC SEA VQIU EXH RZ, RZ UQH

PAHIUHZU HBTHDUREX. UQH PAHIU

FINEARUW GEKH RX EUQHAZ EXGW VQIU

UQHW GHXC QRF, UQHRA EVX ZHGKHZ,

UQHRA KHAZREX ES QRF. -NEQIXX VEGSPIXP

KEX PEHUQH

517. UIHLSLY IWR RODVV DT BJRDA DR HQ ZHHK

GLBNLYWBLTG WTK QDGGLK QHY WVV

GIDTZR. UL BJRG GLWAI BJRDA DT RAIHHVR.

-BWYGDT VJGILY

518. UJH FEJL UJH'GM QE VJNM LZME UJH RDE'P

IDVV DYVMMT SMRDHYM GMDVQPU QY

IQEDVVU SMPPMG PZDE UJHG CGMDBY. -CG.

YMHYY

519. UMYP RDH JVDHDPKK RGP DPYPG NRKWPH.

WTPA RUNRAK SRJP R HVOOPGPDZP. WTPA

CUPKK WTP MDP NTM GPZPVYPK WTPS, RDH

WTPA CUPKK AME, WTP BVYPG. -CRGCRGR HP

RDBPUVK

520. UNUPKECJLH JL AU VUUSG VSTEEUPJLH OLR

VPUU, SJQU J DYTSR EOQU YVV VPYA ECU

HPYTLR OE OLK GUDYLR. ATGJD, J ECJLQ, CU

AOQUG AU VUUS SJQU ATGJD. -SOTPUL

YSJNUP

521. UQK LQS KUG WOS KMWJLYSDSK EOUE WOS

HUW RMSDJS, UQK WEDLQX, UQK RZBB LR

RMDS, UQK EOUE QLE SYSQ WOS JLZBK OLBK

OSDWSBR NUJF NSJUZWS OSD IUWWMLQ

NZDQSK NDMXOESD EOUQ OSD RSUDW. -

CUDF UQEOLQG

522. UQX NREX NRKH, 'UQX DXNU UQKFE KN FJU UJ QRUX RFVJFX, JFTV UJ TJCX. UQRU KN UQX JFTV GRV JWU JS KU. RN NJJF RN VJW QRCX SJOEKCXF UQJNX GQJI VJW QRUX, VJW QRCX EJUUXF OKH JS UQXI. UQXF VJW QRCX FJ OXRNJF UJ QRUX UQXI; VJW MWNU SJOEXU. -QRBORU KFRVRU PQRF

523. UTDQ GJ TH TJCXYHYKFX, LGJDYEFXGHS CQF KYJC KTXEFPYVJ JCTXJ. UFFCQYEFH DQTPPFHSFJ CQF VHGEFXJF. G YHPO CXO CY FZIXFJJ CQF JYVP THL CQF QFTXC YB KTH. -BXFLFXGD DQYIGH

524. UXQTQ RJCQ TIRQH, LXQTQ DH YJ UDRR LJ

NJUQT; SYB UXQTQ NJUQT NTQBJEDYSLQH,

LXQTQ RJCQ DH RSWMDYP. LXQ JYQ DH LXQ

HXSBJU JV LXQ JLXQT. -WSTR FIYP

525. UYV SIUIBV AS AIB WCUFAW EVGVWEQ AW

GBATFEFWK AIB HYFXEBVW RFUY C

HAJGXVUV VEIHCUFAW UYCU FWHXIEVQ

JIQFH. -KVBCXE B. SABE

526. UZNZJH EQR MKMB IMQRFBMJ, UZA MKMU

OZMAR, EZT IFSE Q EMQBA SQU EZYJ. -

WMYJQ DCAWPMBQYJ

527. V CJFR'Z GDZZDJU DZ RJ GVTF SJXHZ HJ

GJXF SJXT REVU REFO UJXGVPPO HJ, RJ

GVTF REFG SJXT JU GJXF REVU JUF PFKFP. -

MVO-Y

528. V UCB WOO NLF NO (WCBYQ GLKMCZ) FLB

AFOBAQ-MVIO SCXOW. FNCA V YLB'A

KBYOJWACBY VW NLF NO HLWA MVIO. -QLSV

EOJJC

529. V UHQQMI HT EHOAVE FJADDMR YXAZEIR VLO

V FMVZZ ZQHHO HL QXI UVQXJHHN ZALE.

ZQJIF BAPEIO WB QXI UHQQMI VLO MITQ QXI

FMVZZ. -N.V. JHUUALZ, QXI QAMQ

530. V XEJW LRIF RX VIN – GMHED, KVJDW,

YVEJNEJP, HNRIA – BVH NBW YRLWI NR

HEUWJDW NBW DBVNNWI EJ NBW GEJK VJK

UEXN MH NR VJRNBWI YUVDW. -IRTWIN

GDFWW

531. V YMVPB HQJVT VP VYJXNG VJ MXENVPC.

VY'J EP XDANSJVLX XDAUXJJVSP SG

MQHEPVYR. VY'J JSHXYMVPC KX EUX ENN

YSQTMXI ZR. PS HEYYXU KMEY TQNYQUX

KX'UX GUSH, XLXURSPX NSLXJ HQJVT. -

ZVNNR FSXN

532. VENSZ SN CR CHIWWCQMW FCIVLRA KLI PFW

FLRLI LK HLJ CRJ PFW GWIVSNNSQMW

JWMSHFPN LK PFW NLEM. -BLFCRR

NWQCNPSCR QCZF

533. VIKWFHKWV H RIMOWA HE KWM CMO RIKWM

AWCSSU VLHF WCPN IFNWA. JWANCJV FNWU

VNILSO SHGW MWBF OIIA CMO QLVF GHVHF

MIR CMO FNWM. -DCFNCAHMW NWJXLAM

534. VJE B ONMXLNO VFMXO NMU PVJI HYMHSY

NVAY SMAYE ONMWY WMJLW. VJE NMU PVJI

HYMHSY LMO ONQMXLN V SMO MG FVE

OBPYW FYRVXWY MG ONMWY WMJLW. VJE

NMU PVJI HYMHSY YJTMIYE LMME OBPYW

UBON ONMWY WMJLW. VJE NMU PXRN

ONMWY WMJLW QYVSSI PYVJ. — WOYHNYJ

RNFMWCI

535. VJPL ILLWI NML ICUTNLIN, GEN UN UI NML

IVJCLIN JT FVV ZSJCNMI. QJ WFQ JS CJWFQ

SLFVVA HQJCI CMFN RLSTLKN VJPL UI

EQNUV NMLA MFPL GLLQ WFSSULX F

OEFSNLS JT F KLQNESA. -WFSH NCFUQ

536. VKL HSG VMLOH HMDG, SG SGULY

OKDGHSMQT HSUH SG IQGJ HK PG DXOMB.

SG SGULY ZGKZRG OMQTMQT. PGSMQY SMD,

UBLKOO EUOH YMOHUQBGO KV OZUBG UQY

HMDG, VLKD HSG ZRUBG SG SUY RGVH, SG

HSKXTSH SG SGULY DXOMB HKK. PXH

ZGLSUZO, MH JUO KQRA UQ GBSK. — RKMO

RKJLA

537. VKTAL AT XGN PIRBKIBN DH XGN TQAYAX. AX

DQNRT XGN TNLYNX DH PAHN ZYARBARB

QNILN, IZDPATGARB TXYAHN. -EIGPAP

BAZYIR

538. VLT CTWBEZ XLE VWGTB VE OGRT NOEZT

XGOO ZEV BQYYTTK NB N LQDNZ ITGZA. LGB

LTNWV XGVLTWB GJ GV KETB ZEV NZBXTW

NZEVLTW LTNWV. LGB DGZK BLWGZMB NXNP

GJ LT LTNWB EZOP VLT TYLETB EJ LGB EXZ

VLEQALVB NZK JGZKB ZE EVLTW

GZBCGWNVGEZ. -CTNWO B. IQYM

539. VNBDY VKCJB UIJ ZJJF BU HUVKILDY – KL

FJKBL DL KFTKGB PJLB UI UIJ'B IJHWJB –

TXDYX DB LXJ BKVJ LXDIP IUTKQKGB. -

UBYKH TDFQJ

540. VS VL IZDXIGOY BPDM LCRDSPVMQ BDVQPL

CM KCOZ RVMI, MCS SC PXFD X LCOY SC

OMEOZIDM KCOZLDYG SC. KCO NMCB BPXS V

RDXM. V SDYY RK HVXMC SPD SPVMQL V

OLDI SC SDYY KCO. -GZéléZVW WPCHVM

541. VS WNR OQEQ ZJJ ZJNXQ VX LTQ RXVAQEGQ

OVLT XN NXQ LN LZJC LN, XN NXQ OVLT

OTVHT LN GTZEQ LTQ MQZRLW NS LTQ

GLZEG, LN JZRKT OVLT, LN LNRHT, OTZL

ONRJU MQ WNRE BREBNGQ VX JVSQ? VL VG

NLTQE JVSQ, VL VG JNAQ, OTVHT KVAQG

WNRE JVSQ DQZXVXK. -DVLGRKV GZNLNDQ

542. VTIH T GLEBM NTVW KFMH KP VOBMH T OHHI DKP T DHO EHTEKFE. CKL OBXX DBFZ BV BE VK VWH EKLX OWTV T OTVHP NTVW BE VK VWH NKZC. -KXBSHP OHFZHXX WKXGHE

543. VUA FIIR HSYA SP SMPNSOAR JT HIEA BMR FWSRAR JT GMICHARFA. -JAOVOBMR OWPPAHH

544. VX FTX FDD F DZSSDX VXZTQ FGQ DZPX'U F DZSSDX VXZTQ, FGQ VRXG VX PZGQ UHKXHGX VRHUX VXZTQGXUU ZU JHKIFSZNDX VZSR HOTU, VX AHZG OI VZSR SRXK FGQ PFDD ZG KOSOFD VXZTQGXUU FGQ JFDD ZS DHLX. -QT. UXOUU

545. VXKUJ GQJHVQ H EQHBQN YLN VQ. HIS U

BQHNIQS ZL BUKZQI DUZE HBB VP GQUIF. U

YLXIS ZEHZ UZ JLXBS DUCQ HDHP HBB ZEQ

QVLZULIK LY YQHN HIS JLIYXKULI NQBHZUIF

ZL VP YHVUBP. -QNUJ JBHCZLI

546. VZWXQ XW WRLNAF XU LZN ELUI-RANV

VAVLND. GSAU GA EATNU WLVARSXUI

RSNLZIS VZWXQ, GA RAUF RL NAVAVJAN XR

ELUIAN TUF JAEXAMA XR VLNA FAABED. -

KLDQA JNLRSANW

547. W DSPT HVT UTDOHWSFEVWR HVOH OFGSFT

VOE NWHV QXEWL... MTLOXET HVTUT'E

ESQTHVWFJ WF XE HVOH WE MTGSFA HVT

UTOLV SB NSUAE, ESQTHVWFJ HVOH TDXATE

OFA ATBWTE SXU MTEH OHHTQRHE HS ERWH

WH SXH. WH'E HVT MTEH ROUH SB XE

RUSMOMDG. -FWLZ VSUFMG

548. W HB EXFJROV XK NLO GXCD. W HB

FXKRNHKNYI FCOHNWKM. W HB H UJRI

MWCY. W YWQO HKV UCOHNLO BI GXCD. W

YXQO GLHN W VX. W UOYWOQO WK NLO

BORRHMO. NLOCO'R KX RNXSSWKM. W

VWVK'N FCOHNO NLO EHBO, NLO EHBO

FCOHNOV BO. -YHVI MHMH

549. W SVWAT PCLRSWLRP QCMUH W CAUZ VBJR

LMPWQ CA LZ CGA SRYLP, QCMUH W UWJR

WA B IYRBS QWSZ, BAH TACG GVRYR W

QCMUH IC GVRARJRY W GWPVRH SVR

BKUMSWCA BAH WAMAHBSWCA CO

LMPWQBU GBJRP, SVBS GRYR B KBSV BAH B

LRHWQWAR. – YBUFV GBUHC RLRYPCA

550. WD RXMMOA FDN UDAAYHM, CAOOSZ, XWS

FOXAMKOEE DYA CDBOAWROWM, DYA

UDAHDAXMTDWE, DYA ROSTX, XWS DYA

AOKTCTDYE XWS UFXATMXQKO

TWEMTMYMTDWE RXZ QOUDRO, MFO RYETU

NTKK EMTKK QO NDWSOAPYK. -JYAM

BDWWOCYM

551. WD SPBT SC KOTK KOBMB SC WXCSN SZ KOB

TSM, WXCSN THH TMEXZP XC; KOB JEMHP SC

QXHH EQ SK, TZP DEX CSWUHD KTFB TC

WXNO TC DEX MBIXSMB. -BPJTMP BHATM

552. WDY OCWKQOG NG YI ESCV INDGOQHOG WCV

QIGO INDGOQHOG WY YJO GWBO YSBO. –

YJIBWG BODYIC, CI BWC SG WC SGQWCV

553. WF'Y JBNL ORFDK GD'SD NJYF DSDKLFEWBU

FEOF GD'KD RKDD FJ PJ OBLFEWBU. – QETQX

ZONOEBWTX, RWUEF QNTV

554. WGMICTVFMJ RLGPV L OMWI IAIC RBGI TIIJOE

QFLC OBAI. OBAI GMVPV TIKICIGLQMCK

MCQB BXVIVVMBC, WGMICTVFMJ MV CIAIG

LCEQFMCK XSQ VFLGMCK. -IOMI NMIVIO

555. WHUMY LJMNBN. CPV YHX OVGQB MB, CPLX

BPLIL HIL IHMXQVCN HXO CMDORDVCLIN,

BPL WGNMY VR BPL CMXO HXO BPL NMDLXYL

VR BPL NBHIN. HXZVXL CPV PHN DVALO PHN

QLLX BVGYPLO QZ WHUMY. MB MN NGYP H

NMWTDL HXO NGYP HX LJBIHVIOMXHIZ THIB

VR BPL DMALN CL DMAL. -XVIH IVQLIBN

556. **WIG PHO WIHW IHWI ON PSUTD TO ITPUGMQ,**

ONY TU ONW PNFGL JTWI DNODNYL NQ

UJGGW UNSOLU, TU QTW QNY WYGHUNOU,

UWYHWHXGPU, HOL URNTMU; WIG PNWTNOU

NQ ITU URTYTW HYG LSMM HU OTXIW, HOL

ITU HQQGDWTNOU LHYA HU GYGVSU. -

JTMMTHP UIHAGURGHYG

557. WIUVHO HTHV LDXXZ, XETH MHTHV ODHZ.

ZQSW DZ UWH TIZU ODAAHVHMSH CHUYHHM

UWH UYE. YWIU DZ ECUIDMHO CB XETH DZ

VHUIDMHO AEV IXX UDRH. YWIU DZ

ECUIDMHO CB WIUVHO KVETHZ I CQVOHM DM

VHIXDUB AEV DU DMSVHIZHZ WIUVHO. -

RIWIURI FIMOWD

558. WMTZ PVR'Z BJKH MN ZDLJRB ZV PV CAIZ

LVM DHIGGL CIRZ ZV PV. CAHDH ZAHDH'T

GVKH IRP JRTNJDIZJVR, J PVR'Z ZAJRY LVM

UIR BV CDVRB. -HGGI XJZSBHDIGP

559. WR'D OC ICCP QYSRSOPWOI RKTR TOG

YSVTRWCODKWQ KTD T ULRLYS WU GCLY

YSECYP ECVVSERWCOD PWDTIYSS

BWCVSORVG CY WU GCLY UTBCYWRS UWVFD

JCLVPO'R SBSO DQSTM RC STEK CRKSY WU

RKSG FSR TR T QTYRG. — OWEM KCYOXG

560. WSGQT VPOC WP KBB CDP GCZPPCG NME KSC

KB CZKSFIP NME UNAP WP GKWPCDQMU

CDNC XNG WQMP CDNC MK KMP TKSIE CNVP

NXNJ BZKW WP. -PEEQP ANM DNIPM

561. WTT TGJS OKWO KWC PGO ILQSPVCKQA IGL

QOC MWCS, QC TQES W NWPCQGP MDQTO

DAGP OKS CWPV. -STTW UKSSTSL UQTRGB

562. X GXF ZSRYQH SIXU X QCMMQI GYZCN [...] CF

RUHIU MSXM LRUQHQD NXUIZ GXD FRM

RVQCMIUXMI MSI ZIFZI RE MSI VIXYMCEYQ

LSCNS KRH SXZ CGBQXFMIH CF MSI SYGXF

ZRYQ. -TRSXFF LRQEKXFK WRF KRIMSI

563. X WCYU LPU AOB VMRXT XJRXZU O TOH

VOIUR BCM QUUW XJYXRXEWU; XQ BCM

KWOB LPU RLUHUC OL VOD YCWMVU, XL'R

OWVCRL WXIU LPU CLPUH KUCKWU TOJ'L

RUU XJLC BCMH YUPXTWU. XL LXJLR BCMH

AXJZCAR, RCVUPCA. -TPMTI IWCRLUHVOJ

564. X'Z VQWYWWYG FXAJ SVZQXYW. X DXTY

FPABJXEK SVZQXY ZVNXYW PEG X HYPG

SVZQXY QVVTW. –TYNXE QPBVE

565. XDA FTDR RGYZ SAWJE JW? CDI'W QJZZQH

VHSJTIHV ZGYZ ZGHVH'W WDSHZGJTC HQWH

PHWJIHW AW JT ZGJW ATJLHVWH, Y

GYVSDTJE EDTTHEZJDT PHZRHHT YQQ

QJLJTC PHJTCW, HLHVX RGHVH, HLHT ZGH

WZYVW. – VDPJT RJQQJYSW

566. XEP FYBA TIO'X XY ATQP UYGPQPG, XEP FYBA

TI XY NGPBXP IYLPXETOF XEBX JTAA. –

NEHNZ DBABEOTHZ, WTBGM

567. XFAT RQFH FGT NTMGJ OF WGFOSTQ PWG FGXZ NT OSWO OCF DFXMOBITD PFHT GTWQTQ, QTPFJGMYT WGI KQFOTPO WGI PFHRFQO TWPS FOSTQ. -SWG DBZMG

568. XFENFP NGOP XTCL, LGIPBPE KTEEGI TKR UEGGHPR, QK ILQUL AGF UTK ITSH IQCL SGBP TKR EPBPEPKUP. -LPKEA RTBQR CLGEPTF

569. XGAM HXGGWHJ! JSUJ CUO JSW CSXAW XL

SWN OWNFXG. XGAM HXGGWHJ JSW KNXOW

UGI JSW KUOOQXG, UGI RXJS CQAA RW

WZUAJWI, UGI SPFUG AXDW CQAA RW OWWG

UJ QJO SWQESJ. AQDW QG LNUEFWGJO GX

AXGEWN. -W. F. LXNOJWN

570. XGNIN CE RYBRVE ETUNXGCOS YNWX XT

YTZN. ROM CW VTK RCO'X YNRIONM XGRX,

VTK RCO'X YNRIONM OTXGCOS. -YTIIRCON

GROEJNIIV

571. **XITKGYB UCYKFKFN KT Y XMCJ RMUJFU KFTUCIXJFU UQYF YFA MUQJC EJGYITJ CQAUQX YFS QYCXMFA PKFS UQJKC ZYA KFUM UQJ KFZYCS RBYGJT MP UQJ TMIB. - RBYUM**

572. **XIWMQ YIJBK WE EP VUPEI NP XIWMQ UPGIK NYJN LPB NYI JGIBJQI SIBEPM NYIH JBI JUDPEN WMKWENWMQTWEYJXUI. -KJGWK JTQEXTBQIB**

573. XJFYUMB F SJFXQSC, FLQUZJ XUOJEQCXJ UE

FXX FDITQ KIKJMQTK. UO U'K UM QSJ

KUYYXJ IO QNFUMUMB UQ'E JFEC OIN KJ QI

VJJW QSFQ TW. UQ BJQE QITBS GSJM U'K IM

F DNJFV." -MFQFXUJ LITBSXUM

574. XJJ HDOBDIW XLH XJWE FHIBDDBDIW. TH

VKWZ OED'Z PDET BZ XZ ZMH ZBGH. - –

GBZSM XJFEG, ZMH CBUH QHEQJH NEK GHHZ

BD MHXUHD

575. XNUK WH C PNZEWOWNZ WZ YBWPB OBK

BCLLWZKHH NM CZNOBKS LKSHNZ WH

KHHKZOWCX ON VNIS NYZ. -SNGKSO

BKWZXKWZ

576. XP NU KSU JB YBEU PBS K OBQXUJW BP

QIRJISKRRW RXJUSKJU EUBERU, DIOXQ DIOJ

GU K MXJKR EKSJ BP BIS QYXRASUH'O

UAIQKJXBH. -WB-WB DK

577. XQN MCSCF PMQU UBWA UQFEC GNZP XQNF

RWO GNZP BWE EWSCO XQN IFQD. – ZQFDWZ

DZZWFABX, MQ ZQNMAFX IQF QGO DCM

578. XSJ WZLJ D XSDOI DX ZUJL, XSJ WZLJ D RJJH

XSEX XSJLJ DQ OZXSDOY WZLJ XLFHA

ELXDQXDG XSEO XZ HZUJ CJZCHJ. -UDOGJOX

UEO YZYS

579. XT RSS JNRQH JRPPT. FL TAE ONG R OAAW KFLN, TAE'SS XN DRBBT. FL TAE ONG R XRW AQN, TAE'SS XNMAJN R BDFSAHABDNP. -HAMPRGNH

580. XTPPTF PW MGET YWETR GVR YWNP, PMGV PW MGET VTETF YWETR GP GYY. -GLBLNPDVT WU MDOOW

581. XZSL BF Q CNWWSG VBKDZNK QU QUFVGH. B'JG CSQAGP KDG XQTG LZH 50 AGQHF QUP B FKBSS DQJGU'K KDG FSBXDKGFK BPGQ ZL DZV KZ CSQA. -XQHA CSQAGH

582. Y FLMH KDCYP. TLX KH, KDCYP YC KLXQYQZ PLTTHH. YR'C KLLE KHEYPYQH. YR'C NDXH KGZYP. G ZLLE CLQZ YC FYBH G ZLLE KHGF – Y WDCR UGQR RL YQIGFH YR GQE RIHQ CIGXH G JYRH UYRI CLKHLQH HFCH. — ILEG BLRJ

583. Y'PK WMSWAI NTEHXTN JKEJMK SEHMF LYZF W MEN CEUK JMKWIHUK YZ NTKYU UEHNYZKI YL NTKA RHUIN YZNE IEZX WN IYXZYLYOWZN CECKZNI. -BETZ RWUUESCWZ

584. Y'V U MLBFI KLI UWA Y'V TUDDI SR XP NYST

STP IUWFPPJ. UWA Y NUWS SR STUWF

PCPHIRWP ERH VUFYWK STYJ WYKTS

WPBPJJUHI. -IRKY XPHHU

585. YBNLW LN PJD QKDRP BOLPDK. RO

LOWKDALCFD EIKWD. NIYDPJLOQ PJRP

HDIHFD MJI ALEEDK IO DSDKXPJLOQ ROA

ROXPJLOQ DFND WRO JRSD LO WIYYIO. —

NRKRJ ADNNDO, VBNP FLNPDO

586. YFO ZS, ICSOS VD DFZSICVHX LOVZVIVGSTW

DFFICVHX KPFAI ICVD ZADVJ, KHB VI USHI

DIOKVXCI IF ZW HSOGFAD DWDISZ, ZKQVHX

ZS YSST ISH YSSI IKTT. -SOVJ JTKLIFH

587. YGPQ WZ CMQ HGZC CQIIWEYQ, JKN JYZG

CMQ HGZC DQKQIGAZ GL CMQ BJZZWGKZ;

WC WZ CMQ GKYX GKQ RMWOM WKOYANQZ

ZGHQGKQ QYZQ. -JYBMGKZQ VJII

588. YKFMC OKXLJ KML VQML ORKE OMSL--EQO

PLBKSJL ORLC OLXX SJ TMKDQEJ LWFJO,

PSO PLBKSJL ORLC OLXX SJ TMKDQEJ BKE

PL PLKOLE. -D. U. BRLJOLMOQE

589. YLUX YDHVD LSF DLWFQ KOZ IF LT QLKF CQF;

EDFS UFQE, SOECUF, ILLXQ, KCQHV, PLBF

TLU LSF'Q SFHNDILU — QCVD HQ KZ HJFO LT

DOWWHSFQQ. -PFL ELPQELZ

590. YN WUR FXOV SUOV YQ WURC SYNV YG JXQ ZXPV RD NUC X KCVXG ZXQW GFYQKA WUR SXJP. YN WUR BUQ'G FXOV YG, QU ZXGGVC IFXG VSAV GFVCV YA, YG'A QUG VQURKF. - XQQ SXQBVCA

591. YVSL DT MEJLIDVI JV YDXL, AVTJLIDVI JV CLMJZ, DEDJDMY VX FILMJDVE, MEC JZL LWAVELEJ VX LMIJZ. -LUDYK CDFRDETVE

592. Z CTQH VHZPM LSAAZHN. ZF'W WT MAHSF FT KZPN TPH WRHDZSC RHAWTP BTX GSPF FT SPPTB KTA FUH AHWF TK BTXA CZKH. - XPJPTGP

593. Z KWIDT RMDEF 1 DEF DV 100 JDHZKU, ZF'U

RMDEF FGK URJK NADNDAFZDW FD MDDXU

NEMPZUGKO FGRF Z SRAK FD AKRO. –IZJ

GRAAZUDW

594. ZFWSV SW BGMLHJC. ZFWSV ZPNMW JMPJQM.

SB VPXXMVBW JMPJQM SX EHCW BGHB XP

PBGML ZMKSFZ VHX. SB JFQQW GMHLB

WBLSXIW. SB HVBW HW ZMKSVSXM. -

ZHVYQMZPLM

595. ZGWW, IS IRLXO ZDL PXNNGKGYJ XY BXFB

LOBMMW; X ZDL LXYFXYF DCMRJ WMTG—SMR

EYMZ, JBXYFL X PMY'J ODKG DCMRJ

DYSIMKG. — WDPS FDFD

596. ZJSUW KN FKBJ MSBJ OJJD NKUQKV, GD VMJ

MSVUJX KN S RGDAVJ. -JXQSU SFFSD LKJ

597. ZPEH MLA ZDSG BP EH: GPC'B APL BNSCQ

APL'IH BPP POG BP ZSCM IPTQ C' IPOO? S

ZDSG: APL'G FHBBHI TNHTQ RSBN ESTQ

YDMMHI. — TNHI

598. ZR Z HKQW EKI ZS CWMYD UW DXMGW SXW

DMCW RMYSMDZWD, SXW DMCW

CMPYWDDWD. -MYMZD YZY

599. ZYMJM XO OFSM PFFE XH ZYXO CFJDE IHE

XZ'O CFJZY LXPYZXHP LFJ. -OIS, DFJE FL ZYM

JXHPO

600. ZYZ LMGVR YCJDU JDAAG XYM DODNXJPVUB

VG YT, KPVAD NYRT LMGVR JDAAG XYM JPQJ

VJ'G UYJ YT, IMJ XYM RQU RPQUBD VJ. -IYUY

Hints

The next section contains one hint for each cryptogram. Find the letter on the left in the encrypted quote and replace it with the letter on the right.

1. U = S	20. H = P
2. A = H	21. Y = R
3. B = O	22. J = L
4. E = T	23. C = F
5. C = B	24. H = D
6. Y = K	25. I = T
7. T = M	26. U = H
8. N = E	27. C = F
9. K = B	28. F = U
10. Q = T	29. W = R
11. J = D	30. U = A
12. C = Y	31. P = R
13. R = K	32. G = L
14. X = K	33. L = I
15. K = E	34. J = B
16. O = P	35. F = I
17. T = R	36. L = D
18. T = F	37. L = Y
19. J = U	38. Z = Y

39. D = E

40. L ≈ V

41. O ≈ N

42. H = U

43. C ≈ W

44. U = O

45. S ≈ G

46. S = L

47. K ≈ W

48. O ≈ H

49. D = I

50. S ≈ N

51. H = V

52. D = I

53. N = T

54. X ≈ M

55. S = P

56. L ≈ W

57. D = O

58. D = G

59. Y = N

60. Q = O

61. V = H

62. F = V

63. C = D

64. X = V

65. F = G

66. P = G

67. K = A

68. G = W

69. D = B

70. J = S

71. G = D

72. G = L

73. D = O

74. I = W

75. Z = L

76. I = M

77.	A = M	96.	C = X
78.	U = F	97.	W = V
79.	T = R	98.	S = F
80.	Y = N	99.	D = U
81.	V = W	100.	Y = J
82.	G = I	101.	W = P
83.	X = M	102.	D = T
84.	M = K	103.	P = B
85.	C = E	104.	G = R
86.	K = O	105.	I = B
87.	Z = H	106.	T = I
88.	O = S	107.	M = R
89.	I = E	108.	S = K
90.	N = M	109.	W = J
91.	A = V	110.	H = C
92.	G = T	111.	Z = T
93.	K = O	112.	G = C
94.	C = P	113.	J = E
95.	U = D	114.	U = T

115. I = E	134. G = L
116. H = S	135. L = M
117. C = H	136. S = H
118. Z = Y	137. O = T
119. B = E	138. A = R
120. S = P	139. C = O
121. X = B	140. B = F
122. N = T	141. U = D
123. M = A	142. U = C
124. K = O	143. H = M
125. U = D	144. R = P
126. O = H	145. W = T
127. Y = I	146. J = M
128. T = E	147. Q = C
129. B = E	148. W = E
130. M = E	149. R = F
131. E = D	150. I = H
132. Y = L	151. H = U
133. H = C	152. O = L

153. C = D	172. R = Y
154. V = M	173. Q = T
155. X = C	174. S = L
156. L = G	175. N = V
157. Q = K	176. O = B
158. G = X	177. X = F
159. N = O	178. D = U
160. Y = H	179. M = K
161. A = O	180. N = R
162. P = M	181. D = B
163. A = R	182. J = B
164. L = T	183. W = M
165. O = T	184. H = R
166. C = N	185. U = S
167. P = N	186. M = T
168. U = E	187. W = M
169. Z = Y	188. X = Y
170. D = H	189. U = T
171. W = J	190. E = A

191. Q = F	210. F = D
192. T = B	211. X = T
193. Y = K	212. L = V
194. J = I	213. Q = P
195. Q = B	214. I = A
196. L = R	215. R = U
197. P = T	216. W = C
198. J = L	217. A = T
199. F = O	218. M = K
200. V = M	219. D = B
201. Y = W	220. N = R
202. G = W	221. Y = T
203. S = H	222. U = W
204. P = W	223. G = W
205. W = C	224. J = M
206. X = I	225. T = S
207. Y = C	226. W = N
208. U = B	227. I = K
209. W = K	228. B = Y

229. U = R	248. F = I
230. U = Y	249. A = T
231. H = B	250. K = R
232. Y = T	251. X = D
233. U = V	252. K = V
234. E = W	253. A = K
235. K = I	254. K = N
236. X = U	255. E = V
237. H = E	256. P = B
238. Q = W	257. W = R
239. J = R	258. M = E
240. O = Q	259. T = O
241. A = I	260. W = P
242. Y = Q	261. E = D
243. A = T	262. F = U
244. E = G	263. R = H
245. S = F	264. F = V
246. T = K	265. Z = D
247. O = S	266. Y = E

267. D = C	286. O = F
268. M = D	287. B = W
269. F = H	288. M = F
270. S = I	289. Z = V
271. B = T	290. X = Y
272. C = D	291. M = F
273. E = S	292. Q = G
274. T = K	293. P = J
275. J = N	294. D = I
276. M = N	295. L = T
277. C = M	296. B = P
278. E = M	297. N = P
279. T = K	298. E = I
280. A = V	299. I = Y
281. W = B	300. X = E
282. W = V	301. T = Y
283. B = N	302. K = N
284. J = O	303. F = E
285. F = W	304. E = S

305. Y = D	324. M = P
306. Q = P	325. W = H
307. E = I	326. R = P
308. G = N	327. F = M
309. R = M	328. T = L
310. H = P	329. D = M
311. R = O	330. K = G
312. K = B	331. R = K
313. B = W	332. C = S
314. B = Y	333. H = M
315. D = P	334. K = W
316. Y = O	335. Q = P
317. B = F	336. O = N
318. T = A	337. T = X
319. D = Y	338. Y = F
320. W = E	339. Q = C
321. U = K	340. N = B
322. G = B	341. W = N
323. H = B	342. K = D

343. J = E	362. R = H
344. B = U	363. R = K
345. L = E	364. H = O
346. P = D	365. E = F
347. H = I	366. L = B
348. J = H	367. W = C
349. O = Z	368. E = L
350. W = R	369. E = O
351. K = A	370. J = O
352. P = B	371. E = Y
353. O = X	372. C = U
354. Y = S	373. V = U
355. S = U	374. A = I
356. X = R	375. A = Z
357. O = H	376. L = I
358. Z = Y	377. Y = Z
359. O = Y	378. H = M
360. G = N	379. Z = Q
361. P = R	380. Z = K

381. C = Y	400. R = M
382. V = W	401. P = H
383. J = C	402. N = C
384. Z = V	403. M = P
385. C = O	404. P = B
386. E = C	405. I = G
387. D = T	406. V = Y
388. J = O	407. U = I
389. U = S	408. J = T
390. A = V	409. Q = O
391. R = T	410. C = P
392. B = S	411. L = B
393. K = V	412. S = K
394. P = G	413. E = D
395. L = T	414. J = E
396. J = R	415. N = T
397. L = M	416. N = L
398. W = G	417. B = F
399. B = U	418. R = D

419. P = T	438. P = H
420. P = A	439. V = M
421. I = Q	440. T = V
422. S = Y	441. Y = M
423. D = O	442. P = H
424. U = V	443. M = E
425. P = G	444. A = L
426. S = C	445. F = T
427. F = O	446. B = G
428. M = L	447. U = S
429. T = F	448. N = W
430. K = B	449. R = B
431. B = D	450. X = M
432. S = F	451. N = W
433. T = R	452. A = N
434. X = D	453. W = O
435. O = G	454. A = Y
436. O = R	455. P = N
437. Z = W	456. V = W

457. B = M	476. Y = M
458. G = W	477. H = N
459. F = B	478. W = O
460. W = R	479. S = F
461. M = U	480. W = O
462. C = S	481. E = L
463. D = O	482. J = R
464. X = F	483. P = O
465. A = M	484. G = U
466. H = M	485. B = D
467. X = A	486. P = H
468. P = J	487. Q = R
469. V = U	488. H = O
470. L = E	489. I = P
471. W = R	490. Q = U
472. F = D	491. Q = E
473. O = I	492. R = H
474. H = M	493. T = M
475. A = N	494. U = R

495. V = H	514. A = U
496. S = T	515. B = U
497. C = J	516. R = I
498. H = C	517. U = W
499. H = E	518. D = A
500. G = I	519. G = R
501. S = T	520. Y = O
502. C = H	521. Z = U
503. R = K	522. O = R
504. T = I	523. C = T
505. D = G	524. H = S
506. I = C	525. H = C
507. L = U	526. Z = O
508. U = N	527. K = V
509. O = P	528. U = C
510. P = I	529. W = U
511. X = V	530. M = U
512. J = F	531. X = E
513. T = U	532. Z = C

533. P = C	552. Q = L
534. A = V	553. J = O
535. T = F	554. O = L
536. X = U	555. P = H
537. A = I	556. H = A
538. Z = N	557. D = I
539. C = K	558. J = I
540. D = E	559. R = T
541. D = M	560. M = N
542. V = T	561. U = W
543. J = B	562. L = W
544. P = F	563. C = O
545. E = H	564. Q = B
546. R = T	565. X = Y
547. S = O	566. I = S
548. L = H	567. C = W
549. K = B	568. C = T
550. A = R	569. P = U
551. K = T	570. I = R

571. A = Y	586. Q = K
572. G = V	587. Q = E
573. O = F	588. U = K
574. C = F	589. L = O
575. P = C	590. Q = N
576. K = A	591. U = M
577. U = W	592. W = S
578. J = E	593. A = R
579. P = R	594. G = H
580. B = G	595. P = D
581. A = Y	596. W = S
582. Z = G	597. G = D
583. S = W	598. C = M
584. L = U	599. X = I
585. K = R	600. V = I

Solutions

1. In the end, it's extra effort that separates a winner from second place. But winning takes a lot more than that, too. It starts with complete command of the fundamentals. Then it takes desire, determination, discipline, and self-sacrifice. -Jesse Owens

2. You want a toe? I can get you a toe, believe me. There are ways, Dude. -Walter Sobchak, The Big Lebowski

3. Perhaps the single most important element in mastering the techniques and tactics of racing is experience. But once you have the fundamentals, acquiring the experience is a matter of time. -Greg Lemond

4. The Russians have a weapon that can wipe out two hundred eighty thousand Americans. That puts them exactly ten years behind Howard Cosell. -Red Smith

5. I like music, she said slowly, "because when I hear it, I . . . I lose myself within myself, if that makes any sense. I become empty and full all at once, and I can feel the whole earth roiling around me." — Sarah J. Maas, Throne of Glass

6. Leadership is a matter of having people look at you and gain confidence, seeing how you react. If you're in control, they're in control. -Tom Landry

7. We can't win at home. We can't win on the road. As general manager, I just can't figure out where else to play. -Pat Williams

8. Chemistry is a class you take in high school or college, where you figure out two plus two is 10, or something. -Dennis Rodman

9. My dad has always taught me these words: care and share. That's why we put on clinics. The only thing I can do is try to give back. If it works, it works. -Tiger Woods

10. **Sportsmanship for me is when a guy walks off the court and you really can't tell whether he won or lost when he carries himself with pride either way. -Jim Courier**

11. **Doctors and scientists said that breaking the four-minute mile was impossible, that one would die in the attempt. Thus, when I got up from the track after collapsing at the finish line, I figured I was dead. - Roger Bannister**

12. **I can't play being mad. I go out there and have fun. It's a game, and that's how I am going to treat it. -Ken Griffey Jr.**

13. **You have to be able to center yourself, to let all of your emotions go. Don't ever forget that you play with your soul as well as your body. - Kareem Abdul-Jabbar**

14. The difference between the old ballplayer and the new ballplayer is the jersey. The old ballplayer cared about the name on the front. The new ballplayer cares about the name on the back. -Steve Garvey

15. My talents lie in a couple of specific areas. He took a mouthful of beer. Looking around the kitchen, Jen said, "I'm betting housekeeping isn't in the top ten." -M.A. Robbins, The Awakening

16. Some people believe football is a matter of life and death. I'm very disappointed with that attitude. I can assure you it is much, much more important than that. -Bill Shankly

17. The Answer to the ultimate question of Life, The Universe, and Everything is...42!" -Douglas Adams, The Hitchhiker's Guide to the Galaxy

18.   It's not the disability that defines you; it's how you deal with the challenges the disability presents you with. We have an obligation to the abilities we **DO** have, not the disability. -Jim Abbott

19.   'Light! Give me light!' was the wordless cry of my soul, and the light of love shone on me in that very hour. -Helen Keller

20.   "...be not afraid of greatness. Some are born great, some achieve greatness, and some have greatness thrust upon 'em." -William Shakespeare, Twelfth Night

21.   "I look into their eyes, shake their hand, pat their back, and wish them luck, but I am thinking, 'I am going to bury you." – Seve Ballesteros

22.   "I wanted to get the fans pumped for the second half, so I sent this tweet: "Need two more dunks on home court for the best crowd ever! #BaylorNation." – Brittney Griner

23. "The most important thing in the Olympic Games is not winning but taking part; the essential thing in life is not conquering but fighting well." —Pierre de Coubertin, father of the modern Olympic Games

24. "When good soccer happens, I give thanks for the miracle and I don't give a damn which team or country performs it." -Eduardo Galeano

25. "You have to do something in your life that is honorable and not cowardly if you are to live in peace with yourself." – Larry Brown

26. "The Greeks believed that it was a citizen's duty to watch a play. It was a kind of work in that it required attention, judgment, patience, all the social virtues." -Timberlake Wertenbaker

27. "Nothing is ever predetermined. It's a constant reminder to work hard, stay focused and never believe that your future is assured." – Tim Cahill

28. "I start early and I stay late, day after day, year after year. It took me 17 years and 114 days to become an overnight success." – Lionel Messi

29. "I always tell kids, you have two eyes and one mouth. Keep two open and one closed. You never learn anything if you're the one talking." – Gordie Howe

30. "His voice was the elaborately casual voice of the tough guy in pictures. Pictures have made them all like that." ― Raymond Chandler, The Big Sleep and Other Novels

31. "Hugh Laurie (playing Mr. Palmer) felt the line 'Don't palm all your abuses [of language upon me]' was possibly too rude. 'It's in the book,' I said. He didn't hit me." ― Emma Thompson

32. "Never give up, never give in, and when the upper hand is ours, may we have the ability to handle the win with the dignity that we absorbed the loss." -Doug Williams

33. "Life is a theatre set in which there are but few practicable entrances." – Victor Hugo, Les Misérables

34. "Aim high and don't sell yourself short. Know that you're capable. Understand that a lot of people battle with a lot of things – depression, body image or whatever else – so know that it's not just you. You're not alone." – Holly Holm

35. "There are certain basic qualities and characteristics you've got to have. Number one: you've got to have a will to win." – Bob Richards

36. "Three hundred and eighty matches a year. And I loved it. I couldn't get enough of it." – Ric Flair in To Be The Man

37. "I became a good pitcher when I stopped trying to make them miss the ball and started trying to make them hit it." – Sandy Koufax

38. "I tell the kids, somebody's gotta win, somebody's gotta lose. Just don't fight about it. Just try to get better." -Yogi Berra

39. "I've worked too hard and too long to let anything stand in the way of my goals. I will not let my teammates down, and I will not let myself down." -Mia Hamm

40. "No matter how much you've won, no matter how many games, no matter how many championships, no matter how many Super Bowls, you're not winning now, so you stink." -Bill Parcells

41. "My nails are broken, my fingers are bleeding, my arms are covered with the welts left by the paws of your guards—but I am a queen!" — Sophocles, Antigone

42. "The hardest skill to acquire in this sport is the one where you compete all out, give it all you have, and you are still getting beat no matter what you do. When you have the killer instinct to fight through that

43. "When I first came on tour, I was playing for money. Now I'm playing to win golf tournaments and the money is more than I ever dreamed I could make." – Annika Sorenstam

44. "Treat a person as he is, and he will remain as he is. Treat him as he could be, and he will become what he should be." -Jimmy Johnson

45. "Every kid around the world who plays soccer wants to be Pele. I have a great responsibility to show them not just how to be like a soccer player, but how to be like a man." – Pele

46. "If one good deed in all my life I did, I do repent it from my very soul." – William Shakespeare

47. "Pain is temporary. It may last a minute, or an hour, or a day, or a year, but eventually it will subside and something else will take its place." — Lance Armstrong

48. "Winning is the most important thing in my life, after breathing. Breathing first, winning next." -George Steinbrenner

49. "I never did say that you can't be a nice guy and win. I said that if I was playing third base and my mother rounded third with the winning run, I'd trip her up." -Leo Durocher

50. "I think he broke his face in the first play of the game, and then he got surgery at half-time and came back to finish the game and they won." — Marshawn Lynch

51. "I am no genius; I just worked hard like my other teammates, and I believe all my teammates can win the title as they work hard, too." - Lin Dan

52. "I've got a theory that if you give 100% all of the time, somehow things will work out in the end." – Larry Bird

53. "If you're using half your concentration to look normal, then you're only half paying attention to whatever else you're doing." — Magneto

54. "It didn't matter what obstacle was in front of us, we'd always carry on to the end. 'Foxes never quit' is the slogan above the tunnel at the King Power Stadium, and we followed that to the letter." – Jamie Vardy

55. "Never compare your love story to those you watch in movies. They're written by scriptwriters, yours is written by God." — Efren Penaflorida Jr.

56. "Hi, you don't know me, but I happen to be married to the man who continues to rudely interrupt you every two minutes." — Ben Ditmars, Ten Minutes in Heaven

57. "Of all the gin joints in the world, she had to walk into mine Casablanca" — Humphrey Bogart

58. "Give them pleasure. The same pleasure they have when they wake up from a nightmare." -Alfred Hitchcock

59. "The way a team plays as a whole determines its success. You may have the greatest bunch of individual stars in the world, but if they don't play together, the club won't be worth a dime." – Babe Ruth

60. "Procrastination is one of the most common and deadliest of diseases and its toll on success and happiness is heavy." – Wayne Gretzky

61. "Every girl needs a bit of whimsy to remind her that life is a game and it's all about having fun." — Candace Havens, Take It Like a Vamp

62. "Movies will make you famous; Television will make you rich; But theatre will make you good." — Terrence Mann

63. "Academia is the death of cinema. It is the very opposite of passion. Film is not the art of scholars, but of illiterates." — Werner Herzog

64. "I got brown sandwiches and green sandwiches. It's either very new cheese or very old meat." - Oscar Madison, The Odd Couple

65. "You're gonna have to go through hell. Worse than any nightmare that you've ever dreamed. But in the end, you know you'll be the one standing. You know what you've gotta go. Do it. Do it!" — Apollo Creed

66. "If I should ever die, God forbid, let this be my epitaph: THE ONLY PROOF HE NEEDED FOR THE EXISTENCE OF GOD WAS MUSIC" — Kurt Vonnegut

67. "Music's always been really cathartic. It's the best drug for me to get away from the everyday pressures just for a second via a good song." – Ville Valo

68. "Don't measure yourself by what you have accomplished, but by what you should have accomplished with your ability." – John Wooden

69. "The mind of a queen Is a thing to fear. A queen is used to giving commands, not obeying them; And her rage once roused is hard to appease." — Euripides

70. "The USA radio frequency (RF) radiation industry has turned zombie movies into reality." — Steven Magee, Toxic Electricity

71. "You can either stick to your goals, or you can just go through the motions and rest on your status. But it's all about work." – Kristine Lilly

72. "Of one hundred movies there's one that is fair, one that's good and ninety-eight that are very bad. Most movies start badly and steadily get worse." – Charles Bukowski, The Last Night of the Earth Poems

73. "I hated every minute of training, but I said, 'Don't quit. Suffer now and live the rest of your life as a champion.'" -Muhammad Ali

74. "I don't run away from a challenge because I am afraid. Instead, I run toward it because the only way to escape fear is to trample it beneath your feet." —Nadia Comaneci, gold-medal gymnast

75. "I'm a pretty good winner. I'm a terrible loser. And I rub it in pretty good when I win." -Tom Brady

76. "The most we can hope for is to create the best possible conditions for success, then let go of the outcome. The ride is a lot more fun that way." – Phil Jackson

77. "There are many Green Dragons in this world of wayside inns, even as there are many White Harts, Red Lions, Silent Women and other incredible things…" — William Henry Hudson

78. "Books and movies, they are not mere entertainment. They sustain me and help me cope with my real life." — Arlaina Tibensky

79. "One of the greatest experiences in life is achieving personal goals that others said would be, 'impossible to attain.' Be proud of your success and share your story with others." – Robert Cheeke

80. "The length of a film should be directly related to the endurance of the human bladder." — Alfred Hitchcock

81. "Music is the greatest communication in the world. Even if people don't understand the language that you're singing in, they still know good music when they hear it." – Lou Rawls

82. "I had seen people fall in love in movies, too, and felt in love from it. And I had seen people die in movies and it seemed more real than death in real life." — Chelsea Martin, The Really Funny Thing About Apathy

83. "I have always tried to be true to myself, to pick those battles I felt were important. My ultimate responsibility is to myself. I could never be anything else." -Arthur Ashe

84. "You can't always control circumstances. However, you can always control your attitude, approach, and response. Your options are to complain or to look ahead and figure out how to make the situation better." — Tony Dungy

85. "There's never any telling what you'll say or do next, except that it's bound to be something astonishing. By God, sir, you are a character." — John Huston, The Maltese Falcon

86. "The advice I will give to my children, if and when they have Olympic aspirations, will be to go for it." —Kerri Walsh, gold-medal beach volleyball player

87. "Ultimately, you have to not worry about people thinking you should have played him differently. You're the one playing the part so it has to be yours." — Ewan McGregor

88. "To say that these men paid their shillings to watch twenty-two hirelings kick a ball is merely to say that a violin is wood and catgut, and that Hamlet is so much paper and ink." -John Boynton Priestley

89. "It's hard to beat a person who never gives up." "Heroes get remembered, but legends never die." –Babe Ruth

90. "The audience knows the truth, the world is simple. It's miserable, solid all the way through. But if you could fool them, even for a second, then you can make them wonder, and then you got to see something really special." — Christopher Nolan

91. "What keeps me going is not winning, but the quest for reaching potential in myself as a coach and my kids as divers. It's the pursuit of excellence." – Ron O'Brien

92. "Who cut him?' Sam liked saying things like 'Who cut him?' It reminded him of being a kid and watching prison movies, which is probably why prisoners talked like that, too." — Tod Goldberg, The Reformed

93. "Focus, discipline, hard work, goal setting and, of course, the thrill of finally achieving your goals. These are all lessons in life." —Kristi Yamaguchi, gold-medal figure skater

94. "Real courage is when you know you're licked before you begin, but you begin anyway and see it through no matter what." -Harper Lee, To Kill a Mockingbird

95. "Most people give up just when they're about to achieve success. They quit on the one yard line. They give up at the last minute of the game one foot from a winning touchdown."– Ross Perot

96. "Excellence is not a singular act but a habit. You are what you do repeatedly." – Shaquille O'Neal

97. "For me, winning isn't something that happens suddenly on the field when the whistle blows and the crowds roar. Winning is something that builds physically and mentally every day that you train and every night that you dream." -Emmitt Smith

98. "Every search for a hero must begin with something which every hero requires - a villain." — Robert Towne, Mission: Impossible

99. "Football is a simple game; 22 men chase a ball for 90 minutes and at the end, the Germans win." -Gary Lineker

100. "Sports teaches you character, it teaches you to play by the rules, it teaches you to know what it feels like to win and lose-it teaches you about life." – Billie Jean King

101. "Nothing is black-and-white, except for winning and losing, and maybe that's why people gravitate to that so much." – Steve Nash

102. "Winning is not a sometime thing; it's an all time thing. You don't win once in a while, you don't do things right once in a while, you do them right all the time. Winning is habit. Unfortunately, so is losing." -Vince Lombardi

103. "I think this is why Ellis took so many moving pictures of us. Because he knew that people come in and out of your life, and a picture fixes them in the moment they reach out to you." – Zu Vincent, The Lucky Place

104. "I've had a lot of drawbacks and setbacks in my career, but no matter what anyone says about me, I'm determined to be the best skier in the world, and no one is going to stop me." – Lindsey Vonn

105. "When I had that attack of pleurosis - he asked me what was the matter when I came back. I said pleurosis - he thought that I said Blue Roses! So that's what he always called me after that. Whenever he saw me, he'd holler, "Hello, Blue Roses!" — Tennessee Williams

106. "Music is a proud, temperamental mistress. Give her the time and attention she deserves, and she is yours. Slight her and there will come a day when you call and she will not answer. So I began sleeping less to give her the time she needed." – Patrick Rothfuss

107. "It is that kind of thinking that is the problem; that movies, video games and the Internet, devices that simply amuse the imagination are more interesting than what a library stocks." — S.A. Tawks, The Spirit of Imagination

108. "Many people say I'm the best women's soccer player in the world. I don't think so. And because of that, someday I just might be." -Mia Hamm

109. "There may be people that have more talent than you, but there's no excuse for anyone to work harder than you do." – Derek Jeter

110. "The time when there is no one there to feel sorry for you or to cheer for you is when a player is made." – Tim Duncan

111. "I've had to learn to fight all my life – got to learn to keep smiling. If you smile things will work out." – Serena Williams

112. "Movies endorsed unwanted ideas by putting them into story form and resolving them up there on the screen. The goal was, as always, identification, but also relief." – Jeanine Basinger, I Do and I Don't: A History of Marriage in the Movies

113. "If one good deed in all my life I did, I do repent it from my very soul." – William Shakespeare

114. "In baseball and in business, there are three types of people. Those who make it happen, those who watch it happen, and those who wonder what happened." – Tommy Lasorda

115. "Pain is temporary. It may last a minute, or an hour, or a day, or a year, but eventually it will subside and something else will take its place. If I quit, however, it lasts forever."– Lance Armstrong

116. "I never travel without my diary. One should always have something sensational to read in the train." — Oscar Wilde, The Importance of Being Earnest

117. "I've always felt music is the only way to give an instantaneous moment the feel of slow motion. To romanticise it and glorify it and give it a soundtrack and a rhythm." – Taylor Swift

118. "I've missed more than 9000 shots in my career. I've lost almost 300 games. 26 times, I've been trusted to take the game-winning shot and missed. I've failed over and over and over again in my life. And that is why I succeed." – Michael Jordan

119. "Bruce Wayne/Batman: A hero can be anyone, even a man doing something as simple and reassuring as putting a coat on a young boy's shoulders to let him know that the world hadn't ended." — Christopher Nolan

120. "Embrace the probability of your imminent death....and know there is nothing i can do to save you." — Suzanne Collins, The Hunger Games

121. "If music be the food of love, play on, Give me excess of it; that surfeiting, The appetite may sicken, and so die." — William Shakespeare, Twelfth Night

122. "Impossible is just a big word thrown around by small men who find it easier to live in the world they've been given than to explore the power they have to change it. -Muhammad Ali

123. "A book is a place where my reality, escapism, hope, despair, love and death lie." — Nikita Dudani

124. "If you're going to play at all, you're out to win. Baseball, board games, playing Jeopardy, I hate to lose." - Derek Jeter

125. "The sportsman has something special inside of him that takes over in difficult situations. I was driven on by the desire, the passion, the feeling, and the pride of being a footballer." – Andre Iniesta

126. "It kills me to lose. If I'm a troublemaker, and I don't think that my temper makes me one, then it's because I can't stand losing. That's the way I am about winning, all I ever wanted to do was finish first." - Jackie Robinson

127. "That's what the movies do. They don't entertain us, they don't send the message: 'We care.' They give us lines to say, they assign us parts: John Wayne, Theda Bara, Shirley Temple, take your pick." ― Connie Willis, Remake

128. "Whenever you feel like criticizing anyone ... just remember that all the people in this world haven't had the advantages that you've had." -F. Scott Fitzgerald, The Great Gatsby

129. "When the mind is controlled and spirit aligned with purpose, the body is capable of so much more than we realize." — Rich Roll

130. "Every time I went away I was deceiving my mom. I'd tell her I was going to school but I'd be out on the street playing football. I always had a ball on my feet." -Ronaldo

131. "I am building a fire, and every day I train, I add more fuel. At just the right moment, I light the match." — Mia Hamm, gold-medal soccer player

132. "I think I'm always so much more happy with books and movies and stuff. I think I get more excited about well-done representations of life than life itself. - Celine" — Richard Linklater, Before Sunrise & Before Sunset: Two Screenplays

133. "I was very against pink and purple when I was young, because they were girls' colors. But that was only because I didn't want people to write me off for what I can do. When I got into my 20s, I decided that was stupid." – Danica Parick

134. "I want to be a dad, first and foremost. I want to be a good father. I've spent so much of my life on the move and travelling around the world that just to set up a home for my family and be a good dad is something that motivates me." – Ricky Ponting

135. "The key is not the will to win. Everybody has that. It is the will to prepare to win that is important." – Bobby Knight

136. "Competitive sports are played mainly on a five-and-a-half inch court, the space between your ears." – Bobby Jones

137. "When I step on that basketball court, I'm thinking about basketball, I'm thinking about winning – but there's so much that goes into thought about how I'm going to open this game up to others. It's so much more than just basketball." -Carmelo Anthony

138. "I could never have gotten back into my career without the undying support of my husband, who works full time at a stressful job!" – Lindsay Davenport

139. "A champion is someone who does not settle for that day's practice, that day's competition, that day's performance. They are always striving to be better. They don't live in the past." – Briana Scurry

140. "My purpose is to go over there and to see if I can keep bringing sports. I'm hoping it opens doors for us." – Dennis Rodman

141. "There are only two options regarding commitment. You're either IN or you're OUT. There is no such thing as life in-between."– Pat Riley

142. "If you asked me what Uncle Vanya is about, I would say about as much as I can take." — Robert Garland

143. "Some people say I have attitude – maybe I do...but I think you have to. You have to believe in yourself when no one else does – that makes you a winner right there. "– Venus Williams

144. "Character, character, character. First, second and third...we were pretty rusty initially. When you have a break for a few weeks you get a bit of rust." – Graham Henry

145. "It's funny how the colors of the real world only seem really real when you watch them on a screen." — Anthony burgess, A Clockwork Orange

146. "It's not what a movie is about, it's how it is about it." — Roger Ebert

147. "Sports creates a bond between contemporaries that lasts a lifetime. It also gives your life structure, discipline and a genuine, sincere, pure fulfillment that few other areas of endeavor provide." -Bob Cousy

148. "Competing at the highest level is not about winning. It's about preparation, courage, understanding and nurturing your people, and heart. Winning is the result." -Joe Torre

149. "I don't have time for hobbies. At the end of the day, I treat my job as a hobby. It's something I love doing." -David Beckham

150. "I think cinema, movies, and magic have always been closely associated. The very earliest people who made film were magicians." — Francis Ford Coppola

151. "Romance is like maintaining a car. If you do a good job of it, you will always have a dependable quiet ride." — T.R. Wallace

152. "Music is all about training in harmony, training to understand and use musical energy for our greater pleasure by attuning to the natural laws of the universe." – Jane Siberry

153. "Books and movies are such different entities that I feel it's best to leave casting to the casting directors. They have a far better idea of what they're doing than I would." — Alistair Cross

154. "Young men's love then lies not truly in their hearts, but in their eyes." - William Shakespeare, Romeo and Juliet

155. "The beautiful thing about it is that no two directors or actors work the same way. You also learn not to be afraid of discussion and conflict." — Ewan McGregor

156. "Ask not what your teammates can do for you. Ask what you can do for your teammates." – Magic Johnson

157. "Keep your dreams alive. Understand to achieve anything requires faith and belief in yourself, vision, hard work, determination, and dedication. Remember all things are possible for those who believe." -Gail Devers

158. "We all come from the same kind of families, that struggled and fought. And if you bring together people whose mentalities and experiences are the same, whose obsessions are shared, you have a big advantage." – Luis Suarez

159. "Human Millipede 6 was the highest-grossing movie of the summer and returned Nicholas Cage to Oscar-winning status." — C.Z. Hazard, Not In The Eye

160. "Film is a disease. When it infects your bloodstream, it takes over as the number one hormone; it bosses the enzymes; directs the pineal gland; plays Iago to your psyche. As with heroin, the antidote to film is more film." — Frank Capra

161. "I love it when you go to see something, and you enter as an individual, and you leave as a group. Because you've all been bound together by the same experience." — Tom Hiddleston

162. "I wouldn't give you two cents for all your fancy rules if behind them they didn't have a little bit of plain ordinary everyday kindness, and a little looking out for the other fellow, too." — Sidney Buchman

163. "At this level, with so many physical talents all capable of doing the same things, the mental side was the separator." – Dirk Hayhurst in Bigger Than The Game

164. "School plays were invented partly to give parents an easy opportunity to demonstrate their priorities." — Calvin Trillin, About Alice

165. "It is not enough to discover the secret of a play, its thought and feelings—the actor must be able to convert them into living terms." — Konstantin Stanislavski, Creating a Role

166. "Fans still talk about my big white scrunchie, which became iconic in its own right. I loved that scrunchie and its little sparkles that Peggy glued on herself. Without my scrunchie, I wouldn't have felt ready to compete." — Shannon Miller

167. "Look after the senses and the sounds will look after themselves" — Lewis Carroll, Alice in Wonderland

168. "What could be worse than being immortal? And still having to behave by the rules?" — Rameau Platee

169. "When you fail you learn from the mistakes you made and it motivates you to work even harder." – Natalie Gulbis

170. "Call me old-fashioned, but The Shape of Water is a tour de force. Maddening. Heartfelt. Sick. Nostalgic. An Ode to Todd McCarthy, Arnold Glassman, and Stuart Samuels' documentary film, Visions of Light. By all means, take a bow." — A.K. Kuykendall

171. "Talent is God-given. Be humble. Fame is man-given. Be grateful. Conceit is self-given. Be careful." – John Wooden

172. "People are less quick to applaud you as you grow older. Life starts out with everyone clapping when you take a poo and goes downhill from there." -Sloane Crosley, I was Told There'd be Cake

173. "Ultimately one has to pity these poor souls who know every secret about writing, directing, designing, producing, and acting but are stuck in those miserable day jobs writing reviews. Will somebody help them, please?" — David Ives

174. "Liberty is too precious to be buried in books. Men should hold it up in front of them every single day of their lives and say, 'I'm free'." — Sidney Buchman, Frank Capra's Mr. Smith Goes to Washington

175. "Take your victories, whatever the may be, cherish them, use them, but don't settle for them." – Mia Hamm

176. "I get nervous about performing 90% of the time. There's always that little self-doubt, but I don't let it get to me." – Torrie Wilson

177. "I think my greatest victory was every time I walked out there, I gave it everything I had. I left everything out there. That's what I'm most proud of." -Jimmy Connors

178. "I train so hard to make sure failure doesn't happen. If I do everything I can, and run as fast as I possibly can and someone still beats me, I don't think of that as failure." – Marion Jones

179. "I'm in trouble because I'm normal and slightly arrogant. A lot of people don't like themselves and I happen to be totally in love with myself." – Mike Tyson

180. "It is rare for people to be asked the question which puts them squarely in front of themselves" — Arthur Miller, The Crucible

181. "Every category has its snobs: music, books, movies. There are so many things a man is only pressured into liking or disliking." — Criss Jami, Healology

182. "I try not to look too far ahead. I could retire as an anchor, but I see myself as always being busy, and I want that connection to sports." – Linda Cohn

183. "I used to think that losing made you more hungry and determined but after my success at the Olympics and the U.S. Open I realize that winning is the biggest motivation." - Andy Murray

184. "I've certainly had periods when I felt like life was winning and I was losing, so I think everybody can relate to that quandary — the temptation to give in, to give up, and then what It takes to keep going." - Malcolm Gets

185. "Show me a guy who's afraid to look bad, and I'll show you a guy you can beat every time." -Lou Brock

186. "I'm not a film star, I am an actress. Being a film star is such a false life, lived for fake values and for publicity." — Vivien Leigh

187. "We are such stuff as dreams are made of, and our little life is rounded with a sleep." -William Shakespeare, The Tempest

188. "Gold medals aren't really made of gold. They're made of sweat, determination, and a hard-to-find alloy called guts."– Dan Gable

189. "There's a time when a man needs to fight and a time when he needs to accept that his destiny's lost, the ship has sailed and that only a fool will continue. The truth is I've always been a fool." — John August

190. "You might not be able to outthink, out market or outspend your competition, but you can outwork them." – Lou Holtz

191. "Love looks not with the eyes, but with the mind, and therefore is wing'd Cupid painted blind." -William Shakespeare, A Midsummer Night's Dream

192. "I just think winners win. And guys who won all the way through high school and college, the best player at every level, they have a way of making things happen and winning games." -Tony Dungy

193. "Float like a butterfly, sting like a bee. The hands can't hit what the eyes can't see." – Muhammad Ali

194. "For me to get through the toughest periods in my life, I had to look within to find the energy to do it. I don't give up. Never have. Never will." – Jonah Lomu

195. "When you do something good, the Argentine people really attach themselves to you. They have so many problems back there that they're looking for somebody to be proud of. I think about that, and I won't forget it." – Manu Ginobili

196. "Becoming a footballer is only the first half of the silent prayer a kid offers up to the sky or confides to his teacher in a primary school essay. The second part is the name of the team he wants to play for." - Andrea Pirlo

197. "It did not last long. It is only in the movies that knife fighters stab and miss and slash and miss and tussle over several city blocks." — James Jones, From Here to Eternity

198. "The principle is competing against yourself. It's about self-improvement, about being better than you were the day before." - Steve Young

199. "I have a theory that movies operate on the level of dreams, where you dream yourself." — Meryl Streep

200. "Soccer isn't the same as Bach or Buddhism. But it is often more deeply felt than religion, and just as much a part of the community's fabric, a repository of traditions." - Franklin Foer

201. "An athlete cannot run with money in his pockets. He must run with hope in his heart and dreams in his head."– Emil Zatopek

202. "Anyone who thinks impressions of old movie actors is funny absolutely cannot be trusted. I think it's like a law of nature." — Stephen King, The Waste Lands

203. "This whole journey was never about making a roster or being on a team. It was about giving myself an opportunity. I wanted to take a risk, put myself out there and put my faith in action. Faith without action is dead. -Jarryd Hayne

204. "Avoid the tyranny of the reasonable voice...it will guarantee a complacency of never trying anything adventurous..." — J. Michael Straczynski

205. "A good hockey player plays where the puck is. A great hockey player plays where the puck is going to be." – Wayne Gretsky

206. "I don't plan on being disappointed. We plan on being really good, and obviously, we plan on winning." – Gregg Troy

207. "I'll do whatever it takes to win games, whether it's sitting on a bench waving a towel, handing a cup of water to a teammate, or hitting the game-winning shot." -Kobe Bryant

208. "Hollywood's Studio Era was part of a Golden Age because it didn't need profanity (unlike reality-television today)" — Manny Pacheco

209. "Movies with interfering in-laws and kids are often presented as comic, the ridicule bringing welcome relief to beleaguered married folks suffering offscreen at the hands of relatives." — Jeanine Basinger

210. "Never marry someone who doesn't love the movies you love. Sooner or later, that person will not love you." — Roger Ebert

211. "The one thing I said all along in the build-up (to game three when the ages of many Maroons players were heavily questioned) is you cannot buy understanding. It either exists or it doesn't." – Wally Lewis

212. "Good soccer players need not be titans sculpted by Michelangelo. In soccer, ability is much more important than shape, and in many cases, skill is the art of turning limitations into virtues." -Eduardo Galeano

213. "You arranged everything according to your own taste, and so I got the same tastes as you - or else I pretended to. I am really not quite sure which - I think sometimes the one and sometimes the other." — Henrik Ibsen, A Doll's House

214. "You aren't allowed back until you've learned to willingly suspend disbelief." — Rebecca Murphy, Plucking Cupid's Bow

215. "I enjoy all the oohs! and ahhs! from the gallery when I hit my drives. But I'm getting pretty tired of the awws! and uhhs! when I miss a putt." – John Daly

216. "I just want people to see me as a hard-working footballer and someone who is passionate about the game." – David Beckham

217. "I was born when he kissed me, I died when he left me, I lived a few weeks while he loved me" — Dorothy B Hughes, In a Lonely Place

218. "Sometimes the things in our heads are far worse than anything they could put in books or on film!!" — CK Webb

219. "We suppress our emotions, edit our thoughts, and behave politely to the point of tedium. No wonder we seek solace in the emotional and psychological honesty of an unfiltered make-believe world of novels, movies, and plays." — Khang Kijarro Nguyen

220. "People want to project their own insecurities on others, but I refuse to allow them to put that on me. Just because you don't think that you could be the best in the world doesn't mean that I shouldn't have the confidence to believe I can do anything." —Ronda Rousey

221. "The worst thing about movie-making is that it's like life: nobody can go back to correct the mistakes." —Pauline Kael, Kiss Kiss Bang Bang: Film Writings, 1965-1967

222. "If chess has any relationship to film-making, it would be in the way it helps you develop patience and discipline in choosing between alternatives at a time when an impulsive decision seems very attractive." — Stanley Kubrick

223. "She is wearing her black dress. She isn't crying, but she never did cry, anyhow. It's a bright sunny day and she's like a black shadow creeping down the empty street." — Jean-Paul Sartre, No Exit and Three Other Plays

224. "TV takes away our freedom to have whatever thoughts we want. So do photographs, movies, and the Internet. They provide us with more intellectual stimuli, but they construct a lower, harder ceiling." — Chuck Klosterman

225. "Then in the spring something happened to me. Yes, I remember. I fell in love with James Tyrone and was so happy for time." — Eugene O'Neill, Long Day's Journey into Night

226. "My parents always told me to be the same person no matter if you're No.1 in the world or No. 1000. It doesn't matter. Always be polite and always be respectful towards others." – Caroline Wozniacki

227. "Worrying gets you nowhere. if you turn up worrying about how you're going to perform, you've already lost. Train hard, turn up, run your best and the rest will take care of itself." – Usain Bolt

228. "At a young age winning is not the most important thing... the important thing is to develop creative and skilled players with good confidence." -Arsene Wenger

229. "There are more things in heaven and earth, Horatio, than are dreamt of in your philosophy." - William Shakespeare, Hamlet

230. "All you can do is be your best self. I'm representing more than just me. I think every person should think that way." – Misty Copeland

231. "I continued to call every week until I finally caught him. I think it's safe to say that this is where I began to learn that persistence pays off." - Justin Roberts in Best Seat In The House

232. "You never really understand a person until you consider things from his point of view ... Until you climb inside of his skin and walk around in it." -Harper Lee, To Kill a Mockingbird

233. "Morris Weissman [on the phone, discussing casting for his movie]: "What about Claudette Colbert? She's British, isn't she? She sounds British. Is she, like, affected or is she British?" — Julian Fellowes, Gosford Park: The Shooting Script

234. "Some soap opera, you know, real people pretending to be fake people with made-up problems being watched by real people to forget their real problems." — Chuck Palahniuk, Choke

235. "Once he heard that books are always better than movies, but he now knew that movies are better than the real life." — Davor Banovic, Girl with Broken Umbrella

236. "You must not ever stop being whimsical. And you must not, ever, give anyone else the responsibility for your life." — Mary Oliver, Wild Geese

237. "Starting with a party scene for 600 cast and end up singing on top of a giant elephant...does it get any better than this?" — Ewan McGregor

238. "There's no backward and no forward, no day other than this. You fill your cart as you go, and that's that." — John Burnham Schwartz, Northwest Corner

239. "When you use more than 3-5% of your brain, you don't want to be on Earth!" -Bob Diamond, Interdimensional Attorney, from the Albert Brooks' movie, Defending Your Life"

240. "Goaltending is a normal job, sure. How would you like it in your job if every time you made a small mistake, a red light went on over your desk and 15,000 people stood up and yelled at you?" -Jacques Plante

241. I'm selfish, impatient and a little insecure. I make mistakes, I am out of control and at times hard to handle. But if you can't handle me at my worst, then you sure as hell don't deserve me at my best. -Marilyn Monroe

242. You like to respect and admire someone whom you love, but actually, you love even more the people who require understanding and who make mistakes and have to grow with their mistakes. -Eleanor Roosevelt

243. The demand to be loved is the greatest of all arrogant presumptions. -Friedrich Nietzsche

244. It is our choices that show what we truly are, far more than our abilities.– J.K. Rowling, Harry Potter and the Chamber of Secrets

245. Early music training seems to shape the young brain, strengthening the neural connections and perhaps establishing new ones. -Dr. Frances Rauscher

246. Music is something that should speak for itself, straight from the heart. It took me a long time to understand that. -Damon Albarn

247. Love is my religion — I could die for that — I could die for you. My creed is love and you are its only tenet. -John Keats

248. Music is a moral law. It gives soul to the universe, wings to the mind, flight to the imagination, and charm and gaiety to life and to everything. -Plato

249. The ultimate lesson all of us have to learn is unconditional love, which includes not only others but ourselves as well. -Elizabeth Kubler-Ross

250. Music? Music is life! It's physical emotion - you can touch it! It's neon ecto-energy sucked out of spirits and switched into sound waves for your ears to swallow. Are you telling me, what, that it's boring? You don't have time for it? — Isaac Marion

251. Clocks slay time...time is dead as long as it is being clicked off by little wheels; only when the clock stops does time come to life. - William Faulkner, The Sound and The Fury

252. You don't love someone for their looks, or their clothes, or for their fancy car, but because they sing a song only you can hear. -Oscar Wilde

253. Keep love in your heart. A life without it is like a sunless garden when the flowers are dead. The consciousness of loving and being loved brings a warmth and richness to life that nothing else can bring. - Oscar Wilde

254. You can't copy anybody and end with anything. If you copy, it means you're working without any real feeling. No two people on earth are alike, and it's got to be that way in music or it isn't music. — Billie Holiday

255. Love is more than just a feeling: it's a process requiring continual attention. Loving well takes laughter, loyalty, and wanting more to be able to say, 'I understand' than to hear, 'You're right.' -Molleen Matsumura

256. A kiss is a lovely trick designed by nature to stop speech when words become superfluous. -Ingrid Bergman

257. I swear I couldn't love you more than I do right now, and yet I know I will tomorrow. -Leo Christopher

258. I'm about five inches from being an outstanding golfer. That's the distance my left ear is from my right. -Ben Crenshaw

259. If being an egomaniac means I believe in what I do and in my art or music, then in that respect you can call me that... I believe in what I do, and I'll say it. -John Lennon

260. Lord, make me an instrument of your peace; where there is hatred, let me sow love; where there is injury, pardon; where there is doubt, faith; where there is despair, hope; where there is darkness, light; and where there is sadness, joy. -Francis of Assisi

261. Anything worth dying for is certainly worth living for. – Joseph Heller, Catch-22

262. **When all your desires are distilled, you will cast just two votes: To love more, and be happy. -Hafiz of Persia**

263. **Love yourself first and everything else falls into line. You really have to love yourself to get anything done in this world. -Lucille Ball**

264. **When you're in love, it's the most glorious two-and-a-half days of your life. -Richard Lewis**

265. **Every thing that you love, you will eventually lose, but in the end, love will return in a different form. -Franz Kafka**

266. **If I can help a kid discover a liking or even a passion for music in their life, then that's a wonderful thing. -Eddie Van Halen**

267. In reality, in love there is a permanent suffering which joy neutralizes, renders virtual, delays, but which can at any moment become what it would have become long earlier if one had not obtained what one wanted, atrocious. -Marcel Proust

268. Neither a lofty degree of intelligence nor imagination nor both together go to the making of genius. Love, love, love, that is the soul of genius. - Wolfgang Amadeus Mozart

269. Love is the virtue of the heart, sincerity is the virtue of the mind, decision is the virtue of the will, courage is the virtue of the spirit. - Frank Lloyd Wright

270. What makes a good book and what makes a good movie are totally different things. –Seth Grahame-Smith

271. To live in this world you must be able to do three things: to love what is mortal; to hold it against your bones knowing your own life depends on it; and, when the time comes to let it go, to let it go. -Mary Oliver

272. What came first – the music or the misery? Did I listen to the music because I was miserable? Or was I miserable because I listened to the music? Do all those records turn you into a melancholy person? — Nick Hornby, High Fidelity

273. Earth's the right place for love. I don't know where it's likely to go better. -Robert Frost

274. Love is the strange bewilderment which overtakes one person on account of another person. -James Thurber

275. The one thing we can never get enough of is love. And the one thing we can never give enough of is love. -Henry Miller

276. Live your truth. Express your love. Share your enthusiasm. Take action towards your dreams. Walk your talk. Dance and sing to your music. Embrace your blessings. Make today worth remembering. -Steve Maraboli

277. Yes: I am a dreamer. For a dreamer is one who can only find his way by moonlight, and his punishment is that he sees the dawn before the rest of the world. – Oscar Wilde, The Critic as Artist

278. Love means having to say you're sorry every fifteen minutes. -John Lennon

279. I love the relationship that anyone has with music ... because there's something in us that is beyond the reach of words, something that eludes and defies our best attempts to spit it out. ... It's the best part of us probably ... — Nick Hornby, Songbook

280. I have found the paradox, that if you love until it hurts, there can be no more hurt, only more love. -Mother Teresa

281. You are imperfect, you are wired for struggle, but you are worthy of love and belonging. -Brené Brown

282. Most of what we take as being important is not material, whether it's music or feelings or love. They're things we can't really see or touch. They're not material, but they're vitally important to us. -Judy Collins

283. In reality, love is about becoming the right person. Don't look for the person you want to spend your life with. Become the person you want to spend your life with. -Neil Strauss

284. Somebody said to me, 'But the Beatles were anti-materialistic.' That's a huge myth. John and I literally used to sit down and say, 'Now, let's write a swimming pool. — Paul McCartney

285. Love is friendship that has caught fire. It is quiet understanding, mutual confidence, sharing and forgiving. It is loyalty through good and bad times. It settles for less than perfection and makes allowances for human weaknesses. -Ann Landers

286. The cure for all ills and wrongs, the cares, the sorrows and the crimes of humanity, all lie in the one word 'love.' It is the divine vitality that everywhere produces and restores life. -Lydia Maria Child

287. I mean, if Beethoven had been killed in a plane crash at twenty-two, the history of music would have been very different. As would the history of aviation, of course. — Tom Stoppard, The Real Thing

288. I love people. I love my family, my children... but inside myself is a place where I live all alone and that's where you renew your springs that never dry up. -Pearl S. Buck

289. When you're making a movie of a book, people are always waiting with their knives. –Joel Edgerton

290. For those of you in the cheap seats, I'd like ya to clap your hands to this one; the rest of you can just rattle your jewelry! — John Lennon

291. If we wait until we're ready, we'll be waiting for the rest of our lives. – Lemony Snicket, The Ersatz Elevator

292. We are all in the gutter, but some of us are looking at the stars. – Oscar Wilde, Lady Windermere's Fan

293. Music isn't just a pleasure, a transient satisfaction. It's a need, a deep hunger; and when the music is right, it's joy. Love. A foretaste of heaven. -Orson Scott Card

294. It's no use going back to yesterday, because I was a different person then. – Lewis Carroll, Alice's Adventures in Wonderland

295. No man, for any considerable period, can wear one face to himself and another to the multitude, without finally getting bewildered as to which may be the true. - Nathaniel Hawthorne, The Scarlet Letter

296. Life is meaningless only if we allow it to be. Each of us has the power to give life meaning, to make our time and our bodies and our words into instruments of love and hope. -Tom Head

297. I believe that a person's taste in music tells you a lot about them. In some cases, it tells you everything you need to know. — Leila Sales, This Song Will Save Your Life

298. I truly feel that there are as many ways of loving as there are people in the world and as there are days in the life of those people. -Mary S. Calderone

299. I don't know (if they were men or women fans running naked across the field). They had bags over their heads. -Yogi Berra

300. As an author, you can't expect a movie to be an illustration of the book. If that's what you hope for, you shouldn't sell the rights. – Bernhard Schlink

301. Love recognizes no barriers. It jumps hurdles, leaps fences, penetrates walls to arrive at its destination full of hope. -Maya Angelou

302. When you are imagining, you might as well imagine something worthwhile. – Lucy Maud Montgomery, Anne of Green Gables

303. Beethoven tells you what it's like to be Beethoven and Mozart tells you what it's like to be human. Bach tells you what it's like to be the universe. -Douglas Adams

304. So many things are possible just as long as you don't know they're impossible. – Norton Juster, The Phantom Tollbooth

305. Music is a talent given to me by God. A medium and a platform and a way to spread a message of righteousness... a message of love, a message of unity. -Stephen Marley

306. We may want to love other people without holding back, to feel authentic, to breathe in the beauty around us, to dance and sing. Yet each day we listen to inner voices that keep our life small. -Tara Brach

307. I'd wear any of my private attire for the world to see. But I would rather have an open flesh wound than ever wear a band-aid in public. — Lady Gaga

308. There is nothing more to be said or to be done tonight, so hand me over my violin and let us try to forget for half an hour the miserable weather and the still more miserable ways of our fellowmen. -Arthur Conan Doyle

309. Twenty years from now you will be more disappointed by the things that you didn't do than by the ones you did do. – H.Jackson Brown Jr., P.S. I Love You

310. What a happy and holy fashion it is that those who love one another should rest on the same pillow. - Nathaniel Hawthorne

311. Love is the answer, but while you are waiting for the answer sex raises some pretty good questions. - Woody Allen

312. There is hardly a more gracious gift that we can offer somebody than to accept them fully, to love them almost despite themselves. - Elizabeth Gilbert

313. Patience is the mark of true love. If you truly love someone, you will be more patient with that person. - Thich Nhat Hanh

314. Music cleanses the understanding; inspires it, and lifts it into a realm which it would not reach if it were left to itself. -Henry Ward Beecher

315. Music education stimulates, challenges, and enriches our young people during their formative, school years; its value lasts a lifetime. - Tammy Baldwin

316. Do you know people who insist they like 'all kinds of music'. That actually means they like no kinds of music. -Chuck Klosterman

317. A lot of guys go, 'Hey, Yog, say a Yogi-ism.' I tell 'em, 'I don't know any.' They want me to make one up. I don't make 'em up. I don't even know when I say it. They're the truth. And it is the truth. I don't know. -Yogi Berra

318. Musical innovation is full of danger to the State, for when modes of music change, the fundamental laws of the State always change with them. -Plato

319. Love is a game that two can play and both win. -Eva Gabor

320. Little League baseball is a very good thing because it keeps the parents off the streets. -Yogi Berra

321. Without music to decorate it, time is just a bunch of boring production deadlines or dates by which bills must be paid. -Frank Zappa

322. Music is the great uniter. An incredible force. Something that people who differ on everything and anything else can have in common. -Sarah Dessen

323. If you aren't good at loving yourself, you will have a difficult time loving anyone, since you'll resent the time and energy you give another person that you aren't even giving to yourself. -Barbara De Angelis

324. I'm already crazy. I'm a fearless person. I think it creeps up on you. I don't think it can be stopped. If my destiny is to lose my mind because of fame, then that's my destiny. But my passion still means more than anything. — Lady Gaga

325. Somebody just gave me a shower radio. Thanks a lot. Do you really want music in the shower? I guess there's no better place to dance than a slick surface next to a glass door. — Jerry Seinfeld

326. Love is the whole history of a woman's life, it is but an episode in a man's. -Madame de Stael

327. Many plays are like blank checks. The actors and directors put their own signatures on them. -Thornton Wilder

328. The book is a film that takes place in the mind of the reader. That's why we go to movies and say, "Oh, the book is better." –Paulo Coelho

329. It is better to be hated for what you are than to be loved for what you are not. – André Gide, Autumn Leaves

330. That's the amazing thing about music: there's a song for every emotion. Can you imagine a world with no music? It would suck. -Harry Styles

331. Eventually you will come to understand that love heals everything, and love is all there is. -Gary Zukav

332. **When you make music or write or create, it's really your job to have mind-blowing, irresponsible, condomless sex with whatever idea it is you're writing about at the time. -Lady Gaga**

333. **I am no longer afraid of becoming lost, because the journey back always reveals something new, and that is ultimately good for the artist. — Billy Joel**

334. **The world is too dangerous for anything but truth and too small for anything but love. -William Sloane Coffin**

335. **The only true currency in this bankrupt world...is what you share with someone else when you're uncool. -Lester Bangs, Almost Famous**

336. **Music is forever; music should grow and mature with you, following you right on up until you die. -Paul Simon**

337. Directing teenage actors is like juggling jars of nitro-glycerine: exhilarating and dangerous." — Stephen King

338. But one of the attributes of love, like art, is to bring harmony and order out of chaos, to introduce meaning and affect where before there was none, to give rhythmic variations, highs and lows to a landscape that was previously flat. -Molly Haskell

339. People ask me how I make music. I tell them I just step into it. It's like stepping into a river and joining the flow. Every moment in the river has its song. — Michael Jackson

340. Color directly influences the soul. Color is the keyboard, the eyes are the hammers, the soul is the piano with many strings. The artist is the hand that plays, touching one key or another purposively, to cause vibrations in the soul. -Wassily Kandinsky

341. To be in love is merely to be in a state of perceptual anesthesia – to mistake an ordinary young man for a Greek god or an ordinary young woman for a goddess. -H. L. Mencken

342. How on earth are you ever going to explain in terms of chemistry and physics so important a biological phenomenon as first love? -Albert Einstein

343. Music is a language that doesn't speak in particular words. It speaks in emotions, and if it's in the bones, it's in the bones. -Keith Richards

344. People ask me how I make music. I tell them I just step into it. It's like stepping into a river and joining the flow. Every moment in the river has its song. -Michael Jackson

345. One ought, every day at least, to hear a little song, read a good poem, see a fine picture, and, if it were possible, to speak a few reasonable words. — Johann Wolfgang von Goethe

346. Love is a promise, love is a souvenir, once given never forgotten, never let it disappear. -John Lennon

347. I declare that The Beatles are mutants. Prototypes of evolutionary agents sent by God, endowed with a mysterious power to create a new human species, a young race of laughing freemen. — Timothy Leary

348. A good marriage is one which allows for change and growth in the individuals and in the way they express their love. -Pearl S. Buck

349. Kindness in words creates confidence. Kindness in thinking creates profundity. Kindness in giving creates love. -Lao Tzu

350. Love as a power can go anywhere. It isn't sentimental. It doesn't have to be pretty, yet it doesn't deny pain. -Sharon Salzberg

351. We can experience nothing but the present moment, live in no other second of time, and to understand this is as close as we get to eternal life. -P.D. James, The Children of Men

352. You create a community with music, not just at concerts but by talking about it with your friends. -David Byrne

353. The most exciting rhythms seem unexpected and complex, the most beautiful melodies simple and inevitable. -W.H. Auden

354. This will be our reply to violence: to make music more intensely, more beautifully, more devotedly than ever before. -Leonard Bernstein

355. I've always thought people would find a lot more pleasure in their routines if they burst into song at significant moments. — John Barrowman

356. It's such a complicated thing to put a movie together. The book world is so much simpler. –Arthur Slade

357. Being heard is so close to being loved that for the average person they are almost indistinguishable. - David Augsburger

358. Let us not be satisfied with just giving money. Money is not enough, money can be got, but they need your hearts to love them. So, spread your love everywhere you go. - Mother Teresa

359. Work like you don't need the money. Love like you've never been hurt. Dance like nobody's watching. - Satchel Paige

360. Life, he realized, was much like a song. In the beginning there is mystery, in the end, there is confirmation, but it's in the middle where all the emotion resides to make the whole thing worthwhile. - Nicholas Sparks

361. He who is devoid of the power to forgive is devoid of the power to love. There is some good in the worst of us and some evil in the best of us. When we discover this, we are less prone to hate our enemies. - Martin Luther King Jr.

362. Love is the expansion of two natures in such fashion that each include the other, each is enriched by the other. -Felix Adler

363. Love measures our stature: the more we love, the bigger we are. There is no smaller package in all the world than that of a man all wrapped up in himself. -William Sloane Coffin

364. Love is never lost. If not reciprocated, it will flow back and soften and purify the heart. - Washington Irving

365. Golf is good for the soul. You get so mad at yourself you forget to hate your enemies. -Will Rogers

366. Flatter me, and I may not believe you. Criticize me, and I may not like you. Ignore me, and I may not forgive you. Encourage me, and I will not forget you. Love me and I may be forced to love you. -William Arthur Ward

367. I know I'm an acquired taste - I'm anchovies. And not everybody wants those hairy little things. — Tori Amos

368. I believe that unarmed truth and unconditional love will have the final word in reality. This is why right, temporarily defeated, is stronger than evil triumphant. -Martin Luther King Jr

369. My heart, which is so full to overflowing, has often been solaced and refreshed by music when sick and weary. -Martin Luther

370. Once we recognize what it is we are feeling, once we recognize we can feel deeply, love deeply, can feel joy, then we will demand that all parts of our lives produce that kind of joy. -Audre Lorde

371. Music is your own experience, your thoughts, your wisdom. If you don't live it, it won't come out of your horn. -Charlie Parker

372. The little unremembered acts of kindness and love are the best parts of a person's life. -William Wordsworth

373. Flowers lead to books, which lead to thinking and not thinking and then more flowers and music, music. Then many more flowers and many more books. -Maira Kalman

374. You've got to be very careful if you don't know where you are going, because you might not get there. -Yogi Berra

375. Definition of rock journalism: People who can't write, doing interviews with people who can't think, in order to prepare articles for people who can't read. — Frank Zappa, The Real Frank Zappa Book

376. Self-love is not selfish; you cannot truly love another until you know how to love yourself. -Unknown

377. If Music is a Place — then Jazz is the City, Folk is the Wilderness, Rock is the Road, Classical is a Temple. -Vera Nazarian

378. Love doesn't just sit there like a stone; it has to be made, like bread, remade all the time, made new. -Ursula K. Le Guin

379. To love unconditionally requires no contracts, bargains, or agreements. Love exists in the moment-to-moment flux of life. -Marion Woodman

380. If I had my life to live over again, I would have made a rule to read some poetry and listen to some music at least once every week. -Charles Darwin

381. I used to think anyone doing anything weird was weird. Now I know that it is the people that call others weird that are weird. -Paul McCartney

382. I don't think you get to good writing unless you expose yourself and your feelings. Deep songs don't come from the surface; they come from the deep down. The poetry and the songs that you are supposed to write, I believe are in your heart. -Judy Collins

383. It is in deep solitude that I find the gentleness with which I can truly love my brothers. The more solitary I am the more affection I have for them. Solitude and silence teach me to love my brothers for what they are, not for what they say. -Thomas Merto

384. When I despair, I remember that all through history the way of truth and love has always won. There have been tyrants and murderers and for a time they seem invincible, but in the end, they always fall – think of it, always. -Mahatma Gandhi

385. If someone thinks that love and peace is a cliche that must have been left behind in the Sixties, that's his problem. Love and peace are eternal. -John Lennon

386. Music expresses feeling and thought, without language; it was below and before speech, and it is above and beyond all words. -Robert G. Ingersoll

387. **Having your book turned into a movie is like seeing your oxen turned into bouillon cubes. –John le Carre**

388. **If you're making mistakes it means you're out there doing something. – Neil Gaiman, Make Good Art**

389. **Golf is the closest game to the game we call life. You get bad breaks from good shots; you get good breaks from bad shots – But you have to play the ball where it lies. -Bobby Jones**

390. **Forgiveness is choosing to love. It is the first skill of self-giving love. - Mahatma Gandhi**

391. **All deep things are song. It seems somehow the very central essence of us, song; as if all the rest were but wrappages and hulls! -Thomas Carlyle**

392. I'm wishing he could see that music lives. Forever. That it's stronger than death. Stronger than time. And that its strength holds you together when nothing else can. -Jennifer Donnelly

393. You, yourself, as much as anybody in the entire universe, deserve your love and affection. -Buddha

394. Magic exists. Who can doubt it, when there are rainbows and wildflowers, the music of the wind and the silence of the stars? — Nora Roberts

395. The minute I heard my first love story – I started looking for you, not knowing how blind that was. Lovers don't finally meet somewhere – they're in each other all along. -Rumi

396. It was the moment I realized what music can do to people, how it can make you hurt and feel so good all at once. -Nina LaCour

397. Music is the one incorporeal entrance into the higher world of knowledge which comprehends mankind but which mankind cannot comprehend. -Ludwig van Beethoven

398. You have to, take a deep breath. and allow the music to flow through you. Revel in it, allow yourself to awe. When you play allow the music to break your heart with its beauty. -Kelly White

399. When you want something, all the universe conspires in helping you to achieve it. – Paulo Coelho, The Alchemist

400. A man is lucky if he is the first love of a woman. A woman is lucky if she is the last love of a man. -Charles Dickens

401. We want a book to be a book. We'll have all the interactive bells and whistles but our intent is to engage young people in reading, not to show them a movie. –LeVar Burton

402. We are told that people stay in love because of chemistry, or because they remain intrigued with each other, because of many kindnesses, because of luck. But part of it has got to be forgiveness and gratefulness. -Ellen Goodman

403. Poetry, plays, novels, music, they are the cry of the human spirit trying to understand itself and make sense of our world. -L.M. Elliott

404. It was sad music. But it waved its sadness like a battle flag. It said the universe had done all it could, but you were still alive. — Terry Pratchett, Soul Music

405. Our lives were just beginning, our favorite moment was right now, our favorite songs were unwritten. — Rob Sheffield, Love Is a Mix Tape

406. It is not a lack of love, but a lack of friendship that makes unhappy marriages. -Friedrich Nietzsche

407. Those who love deeply never grow old; they may die of old age, but they die young. -Sir Arthur Pinero

408. Why can't people have what they want? The things were all there to content everybody; yet everybody has the wrong thing. Ford Madox Ford, The Good Soldier

409. The grand essentials of happiness are: something to do, something to love, and something to hope for. -Allan K. Chalmers

410. Infantile love follows the principle: 'I love because I am loved.' Mature love follows the principle: 'I am loved because I love.' Immature love says: 'I love you because I need you.' Mature love says: 'I need you because I love you.' -Erich Fromm

411. The love of our neighbor in all its fullness simply means being able to say, 'What are you going through?' -Simone Weil

412. Henry Jones: I didn't know you could fly a plane! Indiana Jones: Fly -- yes, land -- no. — Rob MacGregor, Indiana Jones and the Last Crusade

413. We all need friends with whom we can speak of our deepest concerns, and who do not fear to speak the truth in love to us. -Margaret Guenther

414. The times you lived through, the people you shared those times with – nothing brings it all to life like an old mix tape. It does a better job of storing up memories than actual brain tissue can do. -Rob Sheffield

415. The music enchanted the air. It was like the south wind, like a warm night, like swelling sails beneath the stars, completely and utterly unreal... -Erich Maria Remarque

416. Let the lover be disgraceful, crazy, absent-minded. Someone sober will worry about events going badly. Let the lover be. -Rumi

417. We look forward to the time when the Power of Love will replace the Love of Power. Then will our world know the blessings of peace. -William E. Gladstone

418. One can play comedy, two are required for melodrama, but a tragedy demands three. -Elbert Hubbard

419. If I should ever die, God forbid, let this be my epitaph: 'The only proof he needed for the existence of god was music'. -Kurt Vonnegut

420. But I was not in the band, because I suffer from the kind of tone-deafness that is generally associated with actual deafness. — John Green, Paper Towns

421. Love vanquishes time. To lovers, a moment can be eternity, eternity can be the tick of a clock. -Mary Parrish

422. My bounty is as boundless as the sea. My love as deep; the more I give to thee. The more I have, for both are infinite. -William Shakespeare

423. Being deeply loved by someone gives you strength, while loving someone deeply gives you courage. -Lao Tzu

424. Music should strike fire from the heart of man, and bring tears from the eyes of woman. -Ludwig van Beethoven

425. Mickey Mantle was a very good golfer, but we weren't allowed to play golf during the season; only at spring training. -Yogi Berra

426. This song is for the guy who keeps yelling from the balcony, and it's called, 'We hate you, please die. -Bryan Lee O'Malley, Scott Pilgrim

427. A strange art – music – the most poetic and precise of all the arts, vague as a dream and precise as algebra. -Guy de Maupassant

428. I need music. It's like my heartbeat, so to speak. It keeps me going no matter what's going on – bad games, press, whatever! -LeBron James

429. Love does not consist of gazing at each other, but in looking together in the same direction. -Antoine de Saint-Exupery

430. The brains of members of the Press departments of motion-picture studios resemble soup at a cheap restaurant. It is wiser not to stir them." — P.G. Wodehouse

431. When I hear music, I fear no danger. I am invulnerable. I see no foe. I am related to the earliest times, and to the latest. -Henry David Thoreau

432. There are not more than five musical notes, yet the combinations of these five give rise to more melodies than can ever be heard. -Sun Tzu

433. No matter who we are, no matter what our circumstances, our feelings and emotions are universal. And music has always been a great way to make people aware of that connection. -Josh Groban

434. In order to fully realize how bad a popular play can be, it is necessary to see it twice. -George Bernard Shaw

435. Golf is like a love affair. If you don't take it seriously, It's no fun; If you do take it seriously, it breaks your heart. -Arthur Daley

436. I was born with music inside me. Music was one of my parts. Like my ribs, my kidneys, my liver, my heart. Like my blood. It was a force already within me when I arrived on the scene. It was a necessity for me – like food or water. -Ray Charles

437. I never blame myself when I'm not hitting. I just blame the bat and if it keeps up, I change bats. After all, if I know it isn't my fault that I'm not hitting, how can I get mad at myself? -Yogi Berra

438. He took his pain and turned it into something beautiful. Into something that people connect to. And that's what good music does. It speaks to you. It changes you. -Hannah Harrington

439. To live is to be musical, starting with the blood dancing in your veins. Everything living has a rhythm. Do you feel your music? -Michael Jackson

440. Joy, sorrow, tears, lamentation, laughter – to all these music gives voice, but in such a way that we are transported from the world of unrest to a world of peace... -Albert Schweitzer

441. It doesn't matter if the guy is perfect or the girl is perfect, as long as they are perfect for each other. -Sean (Good Will Hunting)

442. Have you ever been in love? Horrible isn't it? It makes you so vulnerable. It opens your chest and it opens up your heart and it means that someone can get inside you and mess you up. -Neil Gaiman

443. Music and silence combine strongly because music is done with silence, and silence is full of music. -Marcel Marceau

444. Music... will help dissolve your perplexities and purify your character and sensibilities, and in time of care and sorrow, will keep a fountain of joy alive in you. -Dietrich Bonhoeffer

445. Love life and life will love you back. Love people and they will love you back. -Arthur Rubinstein

446. If children hear fine music from the day of their birth and learn to play it, they develop sensitivity, discipline, and endurance. They get a beautiful heart. -Shinichi Suzuki

447. My method is to take the utmost trouble to find the right thing to say, and then to say it with the utmost levity. -George Bernard Shaw

448. The greatest degree of inner tranquility comes from the development of love and compassion. The more we care for the happiness of others, the greater is our own sense of well-being. -Dalai Lama

449. A source of trouble is our unruly minds. We can counter that by developing a warm heart. We need to effect an inner transformation, to understand that love and affection are a real source of joy. -Dalai Lama

450. This is love: to fly toward a secret sky, to cause a hundred veils to fall each moment. First to let go of life. Finally, to take a step without feet. -Rumi

451. The first step – especially for young people with energy and drive and talent, but not money – the first step to controlling your world is to control your culture. To write the books. Make The music. Shoot the films. Paint the art. -Chuck Palahniuk

452. Love many things, for therein lies the true strength, and whosoever loves much performs much, and can accomplish much, and what is done in love is done well. -Vincent van Gogh

453. Music enhances the education of our children by helping them to make connections and broadening the depth with which they think and feel. -Yo-Yo Ma

454. Everybody has that point in their life where you hit a crossroads and you've had a bunch of bad days and there's different ways you can deal with it and the way I dealt with it was I just turned completely to music. — Taylor Swift

455. The first symptom of love in a young man is timidity; in a girl boldness. - Victor Hugo

456. You never lose by loving. You always lose by holding back. -Barbara De Angelis

457. We all need friends with whom we can speak of our deepest concerns, and who do not fear to speak the truth in love to us. -Margaret Guenther

458. If you live to be a hundred, I want to live to be a hundred minus one day so I never have to live without you. -A. A. Milne

459. It doesn't matter who you are or what you look like, so long as somebody loves you. -Roald Dahl, The Witches

460. She says nothing at all, but simply stares upward into the dark sky and watches, with sad eyes, the slow dance of the infinite stars. -Neil Gaiman, Stardust

461. Love, having no geography, knows no boundaries: weight and sink it deep, no matter, it will rise and find the surface. -Truman Capote

462. You've gotta dance like there's nobody watching, love like you'll never be hurt, sing like there's nobody listening, and live like it's heaven on earth. -William W. Purkey

463. Age does not protect you from love, but love to some extent protects you from age. -Jeanne Moreau

464. If you develop an ear for sounds that are musical it is like developing an ego. You begin to refuse sounds that are not musical and that way cut yourself off from a good deal of experience. — John Cage

465. I wanted to write and direct movies and not be forced to adapt them from a bestselling book. - Francis Ford Coppola

466. I hold it true, whatever befall; I feel it, when I sorrow most; 'Tis better to have loved and lost than never to have loved at all. -Alfred Tennyson

467. I love you not only for what you are, but for what I am when I am with you. I love you not only for what you have made of yourself, but for what you are making of me. I love you for the part of me that you bring out. - Elizabeth Barrett Browning

468. I play until my fingers are blue and stiff from the cold, and then I keep on playing. Until I'm lost in the music. Until I am the music – notes and chords, the melody and harmony. -Jennifer Donnelly

469. Books and movies are like apples and oranges. They both are fruit, but taste completely different. –Stephen King

470. Popular culture is a place where pity is called compassion, flattery is called love, propaganda is called knowledge, tension is called peace, gossip is called news, and auto-tune is called singing. — Criss Jami, Killosophy

471. Appear weak when you are strong, and strong when you are weak. – Sun Tzu, The Art of War

472. The more anger towards the past you carry in your heart, the less capable you are of loving in the present. - Barbara De Angelis

473. There is a madness in loving you, a lack of reason that makes it feel so flawless. -Leo Christopher

474. Love does not begin and end the way we seem to think it does. Love is a battle, love is a war; love is a growing up. -James Baldwin

475. Movies are not scripts – movies are films; they're not books, they're not the theatre. –Nicolas Roeg

476. Love is more than a noun – it is a verb; it is more than a feeling – it is caring, sharing, helping, sacrificing. -William Arthur Ward

477. Love never dies a natural death. It dies because we don't know how to replenish its source. It dies of blindness and errors and betrayals. It dies of illness and wounds; it dies of weariness, of witherings, of tarnishings. -Anais Nin

478. Music drives you. It wakes you up, it gets you pumping. And, at the end of the day, the correct tune will chill you down. -Dimebag Darrell

479. Why love if losing hurts so much? We love to know that we are not alone. -C. S. Lewis

480. If I were not a physicist, I would probably be a musician. I often think in music. I live my daydreams in music. I see my life in terms of music. -Albert Einstein

481. Music education opens doors that help children pass from school into the world around them – a world of work, culture, intellectual activity, and human involvement. -Gerald R. Ford

482. I think the biggest disease the world suffers from in this day and age is the disease of people feeling unloved. -Princess Diana

483. I wish everybody had the drive he (Joe DiMaggio) had. He never did anything wrong on the field. I'd never seen him dive for a ball, everything was a chest-high catch, and he never walked off the field. - Yogi Berra

484. I'm not saying I'm gonna change the world, but I guarantee that I will spark the brain that will change the world. -Tupac Shakur

485. I've come to the conclusion that people who wear headphones while they walk are much happier, more confident, and more beautiful individuals than someone making the solitary drudge to work without acknowledging their own interests and power. — Jason Mraz

486. I'm always frustrated when somebody makes a movie out of a book and they leave the book behind, or the heart of it. -Sean Penn

487. You learn to speak by speaking, to study by studying, to run by running, to work by working; and just so, you learn to love by loving. All those who think to learn in any other way deceive themselves. -Saint Francis de Sales

488. When we feel love and kindness towards others, it not only makes others feel loved and cared for, but it helps us also to develop inner happiness and peace. -Dalai Lama

489. Never make someone a priority when all you are to them is an option. -Maya Angelou

490. When I am ... completely myself, entirely alone... or during the night when I cannot sleep, it is on such occasions that my ideas flow best and most abundantly. Whence and how these ideas come I know not nor can I force them. — Wolfgang Amadeus Mozart

491. Music has a power of forming the character, and should therefore be introduced into the education of the young. -Aristotle

492. If I am not worth the wooing, I am surely not worth the winning. -Henry Wadsworth Longfellow

493. None of us really changes over time. We only become more fully what we are. – Anne Rice, The Vampire Lestat

494. To be your friend was all I ever wanted; to be your lover was all I ever dreamed. -Valerie Lombardo

495. In my opinion, all men are islands. And what's more, now's the time to be one. This is an island age. -Will, About a Boy

496. The true beauty of music is that it connects people. It carries a message, and we, the musicians, are the messengers. -Roy Ayers

497. Power without love is reckless and abusive, and love without power is sentimental and anemic. -Martin Luther King Jr.

498. To stop the flow of music would be like the stopping of time itself, incredible and inconceivable. — Aaron Copland

499. Information is not knowledge. Knowledge is not wisdom. Wisdom is not truth. Truth is not beauty. Beauty is not love. Love is not music. Music is the best. -Frank Zappa

500. He took his pain and turned it into something beautiful. Into something that people connect to. And that's what good music does. It speaks to you. It changes you. — Hannah Harrington, Saving June

501. To live is to be musical, starting with the blood dancing in your veins. Everything living has a rhythm. Do you feel your music? — Michael Jackson

502. True love is both loving and letting oneself be loved. It is harder to let ourselves be loved than it is to love. -Pope Francis

503. The easiest way to avoid wrong notes is to never open your mouth and sing. What a mistake that would be. -Pete Seeger

504. I saw that you were perfect, and so I loved you. Then I saw that you were not perfect and I loved you even more. -Angelita Lim

505. I refuse to believe that Hendrix had the last possessed hand, that Joplin had the last drunken throat, that Morrison had the last enlightened mind. ~ Patti Smith

506. I'm not going to buy my kids an encyclopedia. Let them walk to school like I did. -Yogi Berra

507. Love sometimes wants to do us a great favor: hold us upside down and shake all the nonsense out. -Hafiz of Persia

508. Music – that's been my education. There's not a day that goes by that I take it for granted. -Billie Joe Armstrong

509. We must all face the choice between what is right and what is easy. – J.K. Rowling, Harry Potter and the Goblet of Fire

510. My music will go on forever. Maybe it's a fool say that, but when me know facts me can say facts. My music will go on forever. -Bob Marley

511. Do you love me because I'm beautiful, or am I beautiful because you love me? -Oscar Hammerstein

512. My new album that I'm creating, which is finished pretty much, was written with this new instinctual energy that I've developed getting to know my fans. They protect me, so now it's my destiny to protect them. — Lady Gaga

513. A religious awakening which does not awaken the sleeper to love has roused him in vain. -Jessamyn West

514. A play should give you something to think about. When I see a play and understand it the first time, then I know it can't be much good. -T. S. Eliot

515. And those who were seen dancing were thought to be insane by those who could not hear the music. -Friedrich Nietzsche

516. To be loved for what one is, is the greatest exception. The great majority love in others only what they lend him, their own selves, their version of him. -Johann Wolfgang von Goethe

517. Whoever has skill in music is of good temperament and fitted for all things. We must teach music in schools. -Martin Luther

518. You know you're in love when you can't fall asleep because reality is finally better than your dreams. -Dr. Seuss

519. Love and kindness are never wasted. They always make a difference. They bless the one who receives them, and they bless you, the giver. -Barbara De Angelis

520. Everything in me feels fluttering and free, like I could take off from the ground at any second. Music, I think, he makes me feel like music. -Lauren Oliver

521. And one day she discovered that she was fierce, and strong, and full of fire, and that not even she could hold herself back because her passion burned brighter than her fears. -Mark Anthony

522. The sage said, 'The best thing is not to hate anyone, only to love. That is the only way out of it. As soon as you have forgiven those whom you hate, you have gotten rid of them. Then you have no reason to hate them; you just forget. -Hazrat Inayat Khan

523. Bach is an astronomer, discovering the most marvelous stars. Beethoven challenges the universe. I only try to express the soul and the heart of man. -Frederic Chopin

524. Where love rules, there is no will to power; and where power predominates, there love is lacking. The one is the shadow of the other. -Carl Jung

525. The future of our nation depends on providing our children with a complete education that includes music. -Gerald R. Ford

526. Nobody has ever measured, not even poets, how much a heart can hold. -Zelda Fitzgerald

527. A poet's mission is to make words do more work than they normally do, to make them work on more than one level. -Jay-Z

528. I can see how he (Sandy Koufax) won twenty-five games. What I don't understand is how he lost five. -Yogi Berra

529. A bottle of Kodiak Grizzly Whiskey and a glass stood on the bathroom sink. Streg picked up the bottle and left the glass. -M.A. Robbins, The Tilt

530. A fine work of art – music, dance, painting, story – has the power to silence the chatter in the mind and lift us to another place. -Robert McKee

531. I think music in itself is healing. It's an explosive expression of humanity. It's something we are all touched by. No matter what culture we're from, everyone loves music. -Billy Joel

532. Music is an agreeable harmony for the honor of God and the permissible delights of the soul. -Johann Sebastian Bach

533. Sometimes I wonder if men and women really suit each other. Perhaps they should live next door and just visit now and then. -Katharine Hepburn

534. And I thought about how many people have loved those songs. And how many people got through a lot of bad times because of those songs. And how many people enjoyed good times with those songs. And how much those songs really mean. — Stephen Chbosky

535. Love seems the swiftest, but it is the slowest of all growths. No man or woman really knows what perfect love is until they have been married a quarter of a century. -Mark Twain

536. For the first time, he heard something that he knew to be music. He heard people singing. Behind him, across vast distances of space and time, from the place he had left, he thought he heard music too. But perhaps, it was only an echo. — Lois Lowry

537. Music is the language of the spirit. It opens the secret of life bringing peace, abolishing strife. -Kahlil Gibran

538. The person who tries to live alone will not succeed as a human being. His heart withers if it does not answer another heart. His mind shrinks away if he hears only the echoes of his own thoughts and finds no other inspiration. -Pearl S. Buck

539. Music makes one feel so romantic – at least it always gets on one's nerves – which is the same thing nowadays. -Oscar Wilde

540. It is dreadful when something weighs on your mind, not to have a soul to unburden yourself to. You know what I mean. I tell my piano the things I used to tell you. - Frédéric Chopin

541. If you were all alone in the universe with no one to talk to, no one with which to share the beauty of the stars, to laugh with, to touch, what would be your purpose in life? It is other life, it is love, which gives your life meaning. -Mitsugi Saotome

542. Take a music bath once or twice a week for a few seasons. You will find it is to the soul what a water bath is to the body. -Oliver Wendell Holmes

543. The good life is inspired by love and guided by knowledge. -Bertrand Russell

544. We are all a little weird and life's a little weird, and when we find someone whose weirdness is compatible with ours, we join up with them and fall in mutual weirdness and call it love. -Dr. Seuss

545. Music became a healer for me. And I learned to listen with all my being. I found that it could wipe away all the emotions of fear and confusion relating to my family. -Eric Clapton

546. Music is stored in our long-term memory. When we learn something through music, we tend to remember it longer and believe it more deeply. -Joyce Brothers

547. I love the relationship that anyone has with music... because there's something in us that is beyond the reach of words, something that eludes and defies our best attempts to spit it out. It's the best part of us probably. -Nick Hornby

548. I am focused on the work. I am constantly creating. I am a busy girl. I live and breathe my work. I love what I do. I believe in the message. There's no stopping. I didn't create the fame, the fame created me. - Lady Gaga

549. I think sometimes could I only have music on my own terms, could I live in a great city, and know where I could go whenever I wished the ablution and inundation of musical waves, that were a bath and a medicine. – Ralph Waldo Emerson

550. No matter how corrupt, greedy, and heartless our government, our corporations, our media, and our religious and charitable institutions may become, the music will still be wonderful. -Kurt Vonnegut

551. My idea is that there is music in the air, music all around us; the world is full of it, and you simply take as much as you require. -Edward Elgar

552. Art enables us to find ourselves and lose ourselves at the same time. – Thomas Merton, No Man Is an Island

553. It's only after we've lost everything that we're free to do anything. – Chuck Palahniuk, Fight Club

554. Friendship marks a life even more deeply than love. Love risks degenerating into obsession, friendship is never anything but sharing. -Elie Wiesel

555. Magic exists. Who can doubt it, when there are rainbows and wildflowers, the music of the wind and the silence of the stars. Anyone who has loved has been touched by magic. It is such a simple and such an extraordinary part of the lives we live. -Nora Roberts

556. The man that hath no music in himself, nor is not moved with concord of sweet sounds, is fit for treasons, stratagems, and spoils; the motions of his spirit are dull as night, and his affections dark as Erebus. -William Shakespeare

557. Hatred ever kills, love never dies. Such is the vast difference between the two. What is obtained by love is retained for all time. What is obtained by hatred proves a burden in reality for it increases hatred. -Mahatma Gandhi

558. Just don't give up trying to do what you really want to do. Where there's love and inspiration, I don't think you can go wrong. -Ella Fitzgerald

559. It's no good pretending that any relationship has a future if your record collections disagree violently or if your favorite films wouldn't even speak to each other if they met at a party. — Nick Hornby

560. Music kept me off the streets and out of trouble and gave me something that was mine that no one could take away from me. -Eddie Van Halen

561. All love that has not friendship for its base, is like a mansion built upon the sand. -Ella Wheeler Wilcox

562. A man should hear a little music [...] in order that worldly cares may not obliterate the sense of the beautiful which God has implanted in the human soul. -Johann Wolfgang von Goethe

563. I love the way music inside a car makes you feel invisible; if you play the stereo at max volume, it's almost like the other people can't see into your vehicle. It tints your windows, somehow. -Chuck Klosterman

564. I'm obsessed with zombies. I like watching zombie movies and I read zombie books. –Kevin Bacon

565. You know what music is? God's little reminder that there's something else besides us in this universe, a harmonic connection between all living beings, every where, even the stars. – Robin Williams

566. The goal isn't to live forever, the goal is to create something that will. – Chuck Palahniuk, Diary

567. Love from one being to another can only be that two solitudes come nearer, recognize and protect and comfort each other. -Han Suyin

568. Pursue some path, however narrow and crooked, in which you can walk with love and reverence. -Henry David Thoreau

569. Only connect! That was the whole of her sermon. Only connect the prose and the passion, and both will be exalted, and human love will be seen at its height. Live in fragments no longer. -E. M. Forster

570. **There is always something left to love. And if you ain't learned that, you ain't learned nothing. -Lorraine Hansberry**

571. **Musical training is a more potent instrument than any other because rhythm and harmony find their way into the inward places of the soul. - Plato**

572. **Being heard is so close to being loved that for the average person they are almost indistinguishable. - David Augsburger**

573. **Leading a healthy, active lifestyle is all about momentum. If I'm in the middle of training it's easy for me to keep that up. It gets tough when I'm on a break." -Natalie Coughlin**

574. **All endings are also beginnings. We just don't know it at the time. - Mitch Albom, The Five People You Meet in Heaven**

575. Love is a condition in which the happiness of another person is essential to your own. -Robert Heinlein

576. If we are to hope for a society of culturally literate people, music must be a vital part of our children's education. -Yo-Yo Ma

577. You never know what worse luck your bad luck has saved you from. – Cormac McCarthy, No Country For Old Men

578. The more I think it over, the more I feel that there is nothing more truly artistic than to love people. -Vincent van Gogh

579. By all means marry. If you get a good wife, you'll be happy. If you get a bad one, you'll become a philosopher. -Socrates

580. Better to have loved and lost, than to have never loved at all. - Augustine of Hippo

581. Golf is a puzzle without an answer. I've played the game for 50 years and I still haven't the slightest idea of how to play. -Gary Player

582. I love music. For me, music is morning coffee. It's mood medicine. It's pure magic. A good song is like a good meal – I just want to inhale it and then share a bite with someone else. — Hoda Kotb

583. I've always thought people would find a lot more pleasure in their routines if they burst into song at significant moments. -John Barrowman

584. I'm a lucky guy and I'm happy to be with the Yankees. And I want to thank everyone for making this night necessary. -Yogi Berra

585. Music is the great uniter. An incredible force. Something that people who differ on everything and anything else can have in common. — Sarah Dessen, Just Listen

586. For me, there is something primitively soothing about this music, and it went straight to my nervous system, making me feel ten feet tall. -Eric Clapton

587. Love is the most terrible, and also the most generous of the passions; it is the only one which includes in its dreams the happiness of someone else. -Alphonse Karr

588. Fairy tales are more than true--not because they tell us dragons exist, but because they tell us dragons can be beaten. -G. K. Chesterton

589. Work which one hopes may be of some use; then rest, nature, books, music, love for one's neighbor — such is my idea of happiness. -Leo Tolstoy

590. If you have love in your life it can make up for a great many things you lack. If you don't have it, no matter what else there is, it's not enough. -Ann Landers

591. Love is anterior to life, posterior to death, initial of creation, and the Exponent of earth. -Emily Dickinson

592. I love being married. It's so great to find one special person you want to annoy for the rest of your life. -Unknown

593. I enjoy about 1 out of 100 movies, it's about the same proportion to books published that I care to read. –Jim Harrison

594. Music is therapy. Music moves people. It connects people in ways that no other medium can. It pulls heart strings. It acts as medicine. -Macklemore

595. Well, my music was different in high school; I was singing about love— you know, things I don't care about anymore. — Lady Gaga

596. Years of love have been forgot, in the hatred of a minute. -Edgar Allan Poe

597. Some guy said to me: Don't you think you're too old to sing rock n' roll? I said: You'd better check with Mick Jagger. — Cher

598. If I love you it means we share the same fantasies, the same madnesses. -Anais Nin

599. There is some good in this world and it's worth fighting for. -Sam, Lord of the Rings

600. Pop music often tells you everything is OK, while rock music tells you that it's not OK, but you can change it. -Bono

Find more of our puzzle books where you bought this one. Cryptograms, Sudoku, and much more.

For a free Sample Pack of puzzles, sign up at https://www.subscribepage.com/samplepack

Made in the USA
Coppell, TX
03 January 2024

27168098R00227